The Dermatologist's Guide to Looking Younger

The Dermatologist's Guide to Looking Younger

By Lawrence J. Green, M.D.

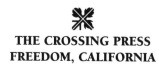

THE CROSSING PRESS
FREEDOM, CALIFORNIA

This book is not intended to replace the services of a licensed health care provider in the diagnosis or treatment of illness, disease, or condition. Any application of the material set forth in this book is at the reader's discretion and sole responsibility.

Copyright © 1999 by Lawrence J. Green, M.D.
Cover design by Victoria May
Cover photograph by Myra Miller
Printed in the U.S.A.

For information on bulk purchases or group discounts for this and other Crossing Press titles, please contact our Special Sales Manager at 800/777-1048.
Visit our Web site: **www.crossingpress.com**

Library of Congress Cataloging-in-Publication Data

Green, Lawrence J.
    The dermatologist's guide to looking younger / by Lawrence J. Green.
        p. cm.
    ISBN 0-89594-952-0
    1. Skin—Care and hygiene—Encyclopedias. 2. Skin—Aging—Prevention—Encyclopedias. I. Title.
RL87.G685   1999
616.5—dc21   98-55321
                                                CIP

Acknowledgments

I am sincerely grateful to all of the following people, because without them writing this book would have been impossible. I must first thank Andy Cohen, a film producer in Los Angeles, whose invaluable contribution cannot be overestimated.

Ednan Mushtaq, M.D., a facial plastic surgeon in Falls Church, Virginia, was instrumental in providing me with information on facial plastic procedures, and took the time to review these relevant entries. Dr. Mushtaq and I have a long working relationship since our training in Southern California. Anne Nickodem, M.D., a plastic surgeon in Fairfax, Virginia, also helped provide information on plastic surgery procedures. I used the expertise of Brenda Dintiman, M.D., a dermatologist, and Debbie Melvin-Unthank, an aesthetician, both in Fairfax, Virginia, to assist with some of the entries pertaining to diet and makeup, respectively. Jeffrey Rodney, D.M.D., a cosmetic, restorative dentist in Pennington, New Jersey, helped write and edit the entry on teeth, truly showing how much of an expert he is in his field.

Most important, I would like to thank my parents, Leonard and Adele Green, whose critical reading and excellent editing suggestions made this book a more reader-friendly guide. I can never thank them enough for their support, time, and dedication to this project. My in-laws, Barbara and Bob Frager, also provided much emotional support.

And finally, my wife Allison, to whom this book is dedicated, I wish to thank for being the best, most supportive spouse anyone can imagine. She endured countless hours of my writing, and then herself spent countless hours helping edit the manuscript. She, along with my daughter Yael, truly is my source of happiness.

Introduction

I began thinking about this book a few years ago when I spoke about a new wrinkle cream on a local TV program. A famous author who was on the same program came over afterwards to thank me for my simple, straightforward answers. She had searched high and low for an answer to a skin problem, but got nowhere. She suggested that I write a book to help other women who needed clear information about aging skin. At first I did not take her suggestion seriously, but when several other women approached me with similar requests, I listened and accepted the fact that there was a need for such a book. I began to realize that, during the last fifteen years so many anti-aging remedies have appeared on the market, it is almost impossible for people to sort through them. I have attempted to fill this gap and hope you find this book helpful. It is not meant to be a substitute for a physician's advice, but only to educate you about what's available in the marketplace today. If you wish to go further, you should see a dermatologist or a plastic surgeon in order to decide what methods are best for you.

A

Aging

From the moment we are born we start to age. No one really knows why we have to age but there are two popular theories. One of these theories focuses on our bodies' decreasing ability to stop dangerous free radicals from destroying our cells. (Free radicals are toxic molecules formed from things such as air pollution, smoking, and exposure to sun.) Instead of our cells dying from outside forces such as free radicals, another theory hypothesizes an internal cause. The protective tips of our genetic-rich chromosomes, called telomeres, progressively shorten each time a cell divides. When telomeres become too short, the chromosomes cannot work properly and the cells eventually die. Because our cells, the very life form of our bodies, are finite, so are our bodies.

No matter what the cause, the ravages of aging are seen on our faces and bodies. After several decades of life, our skin becomes thinner and less resilient. Gravity also takes its toll and what was firm skin starts to sag. Even our mouths are less firm, and the corners of our mouths turn downward. Crossing lines on our faces, also known as sleep lines, hatch and cross each other. These lines seem to be more noticeable on men's foreheads and women's cheeks. Years of smiling and frowning carve their own lines into our skin.

And years of sun exposure accumulate and contribute to the most visible effects of facial aging, a process dermatologists refer to as "photoaging." Photoaging makes our wrinkles deeper, our skin rough and leathery, and our coloring brown and blotchy. Photoaging adds tiny, fine blood vessels to our skin and contributes to possible precancerous and cancerous growths. Sun-damaged, or photoaged, skin is what we use to gauge how old someone is.

Dermatologists and facial plastic surgeons help make your face look younger by hiding all of these features of aging. Think about it: a baby's face is soft and smooth and the cheek, jaw, chin, forehead, and nose all blend together into one. The eyes and mouth are most prominent. Not surprisingly, glamorous models also have prominent eyes and lips, and the rest of their faces harmoniously supports these features. Dermatologists and facial plastic surgeons can help you look more youthful by smoothing, filling in, relaxing, or tightening up your skin—all of which work to restore a more harmonious, blended appearance. Further details on methods used to reverse the aging process are presented throughout the book.

See also: Collagen, chemical peels, face-lifts, intrinsic aging, lasers, photoaging, wrinkles

Alexandrite *[al-eggs-an-drite]* laser

The Alexandrite laser is a laser that removes natural and unnatural pigmentation, such as tattoos. Named after the Alexandrite crystal—which gives this laser its unique corrective properties—the Alexandrite laser shoots the skin with pulses of concentrated light energy that is visible to the eye as the color red. The laser's miniscule wavelength passes through the skin and then strikes the pigmented cells underneath the skin's surface and obliterates them. This procedure can help lighten sun freckles, skin discoloration such as melasma, and the pigmentation that sometimes follows a rash that has faded. The Alexandrite laser is not used for skin repair.

In addition, this laser effectively removes unwanted hair. When used properly, it can target pigment cells in the hair near the area where hair growth begins, and thereby destroy the hair at its root.

Similar to other lasers, the Alexandrite carries a small risk of leaving a pigmented mark at the target site. Darker-skinned people are at higher risk. If a "cooling tip" is added to an Alexandrite laser there will be a large decrease in pain and side effects. Consult your dermatologist for possible risks.

See also: Neodymium:Yag laser, mask of pregnancy, melasma

Alloderm *[al-o-derm]*

Alloderm is a collagen-like substance that is used to fill in cracks or deep wrinkles of the skin. Alloderm is made from skin taken from a human skin bank, which is then processed to remove everything but the collagen, a skin protein. Technicians dissolve the skin cells with salts and detergents and then dehydrate it to leave essentially pure, human-derived collagen. Alloderm comes in millimeter-thin sheets that your doctor shapes and then implants under your skin using minute incisions so that the wrinkles are filled with the material.

Alloderm can be shaped to fill deeper wrinkles. Another wrinkle-filler, Gore-Tex, may be used for the same problem. Alloderm can be applied to the lips (to gain fuller lips) and to the deep creases that often separate the cheeks from the mouth. Alloderm also helps repair scars. Alloderm is available in many dermatologists' and plastic surgeons' offices as a simple outpatient procedure. Because Alloderm is derived from human skin and not cow's skin (the base for the brand name Collagen), the risk of allergic reaction is virtually nonexistent.

See also: Autologen, Collagen, fat transplantation, Gore-Tex

Alphahydroxy *[al-fa-hie-drox-ee]* acids

Alphahydroxy acids are derived from a variety of sources, including sugarcane, milk, and fruit.

Refined by chemist Eugene Van Scott, Ph.D., in the 1970s, these mild, natural acids improve the look and feel of skin by gently removing the dead skin cells and possibly regenerating collagen. Dr. Van Scott's discovery failed to interest physicians during the 1970s and 1980s. In the 1990s when Retin-A became recognized as a rejuvenating agent, dermatologists realized that the alphahydroxy acids might be useful for wrinkles. (Retin-A is an acne medicine that also happens to reduce fine wrinkles.)

It is likely that the antiaging effects of alphahydroxy acids were known in the ancient world. Twenty centuries before Dr. Van Scott was born, Cleopatra was supposed to have bathed in fermented wines (that contained alphahydroxy acids) in order to maintain her youthful glow. Ancient Egyptians were also reported to have used sour milk (which contains the alphahydroxy acid, lactic acid) to keep their skin softer.

Today the two most commonly used alphahydroxy acids are glycolic acid and lactic acid. (Glycolic acid has the better track record.) Topical agents of these acids are available over the counter, while prescription-strength agents may be purchased at your dermatologist's office. Over-the-counter alphahydroxy acids are available in a pure form or in combination with moisturizers. These help exfoliate your skin and make it youthful looking. Over-the-counter glycolic acids generally contain less than 10 percent "free" glycolic acid (the amount of acid immediately available to work directly on your skin). Prescription-strength glycolic acids generally contain more than 10 percent free acid concentration.

Some studies suggest that the stronger alphahydroxy acid products prescribed by dermatologists increase the flow of blood to your skin and help create new skin cells and collagen. This growth of new skin cells and new collagen helps improve sun-damaged skin beyond the mere exfoliation effected by over-the-counter alphahydroxy acids. After several months of application, prescription alphahydroxy acids can reduce wrinkles and brown, blotchy spots. These acids can also be used with the anti-wrinkle cream Renova to achieve an even greater reduction of sun damage.

How do alphahydroxy acids compare to Renova? Consistent application of alphahydroxy acids will improve the look of your skin; however, today most dermatologists believe that they are less effective than Renova; that the daily use of topical, prescription-strength glycolic acid is roughly about half as effective as the daily use of Renova. Alphahydroxy acids and Renova can be used together for better effect—provided they are applied at different times of the day.

Glycolic acid is also available in superficial chemical peels, sometimes called "lunchtime peels," in salons and in prescription strength at your dermatologist's office. Salon peels are not as strong as those applied at a dermatologist's office. While peels are much stronger than lotions and creams (with the same ingredient) applied daily, their effects lessen after a few weeks unless they are repeated. A daily regimen of skin rejuvenation products such as alphahydroxy acids or Renova enhances the effect of these peels.

See also: Betahydroxy acids, fine wrinkles, glycolic acid, lactic acid, Renova, sun damage, sun freckles

Amniotic *[am-nee-au-tik]* fluid

Amniotic fluid is sold as a topical cosmetic application to increase cell growth. Derived from cow fetuses, the amniotic fluid is extracted from pregnant cows and then packaged in both moisturizer and compound form and sold over the counter. It is also an ingredient in certain face moisturizers, hair lotions, and breast-firming creams.

Theories that support its topical application say that amniotic fluid penetrates the skin and spurs cells on to grow faster; however, this theory has yet to be proven scientifically. Therefore, most dermatologists and other skin-care practitioners do not acknowledge this fluid as an effective remedy. Despite its lack of medical support, over-the-counter skin-care products containing this fluid continue to sell.

See also: Placenta extract

Antioxidants *[an-tie-ox-e-dents]*
Antioxidants are compounds that may help us look and feel younger. Antioxidants can be taken as pills or applied topically to the skin. When taken orally, they circulate throughout the body, while topically applied antioxidants work primarily on the surface of the skin. Common antioxidants are vitamin C, vitamin E, the enzyme catalase, the enzyme superoxide dismutase, and beta-carotene, a form of vitamin A. All of these antioxidants are available over the counter in pill form; vitamins C and E are available also in topical form.

When applied to your skin or taken orally, antioxidants lessen or eliminate the harmful effects of free radicals, molecules that are stimulated and therefore multiply when sun rays strike your skin. Free radicals are unstable because they have unpaired electrons: one free radical can readily trigger the formation of thousands of additional, havoc-wreaking free radicals. Because they are inherent in the sun's rays and the polluted air, it is hard to avoid coming into contact with them.

Because antioxidants help rid your skin of free radicals, dermatologists call this action a "quenching." In other words, antioxidants provide free radicals with a stable home so that they no longer rumble around your skin wreaking havoc and potentially leading to cancer. Much of the current research involves harvesting antioxidants from plants and plant materials such as leaves, bark, and seeds. Though scientific research in this area is in its infancy, it seems to be likely that antioxidants are beneficial to our health.

Vitamins C and E taken together as pills are known to slightly decrease sunburn. Topical antioxidants may also help prevent further photoaging of the skin (photoaging is what causes wrinkles and is a sign of sun damage), especially when applied at the same time as a sunscreen. The media has begun paying attention to antioxidants because of their potential restorative qualities and contribution to preventative health.

It may be that the best way to enhance your health is to eat plenty of fresh fruits and vegetables and to consider taking vitamin supplements. Consult your doctor for the supplements best for you.

See also: Free radicals, sun damage, vitamin A, vitamin C, vitamin E

Artecoll

Artecoll is a wrinkle-filling substance that has been used in Europe for a number of years, but is currently awaiting approval by the FDA for use in the United States. Through breakthroughs in microtechnology, Artecoll implants contain Collagen combined with microspheres (microscopic fillers that adhere to the Collagen). (Collagen is the trade name for animal-derived collagen especially treated to replace the biological collagen in your skin.) Artecoll's microspheres are made of a safe, synthetic material that, combined with Collagen, smoothes out your skin.

Here's how Artecoll is supposed to work. Your dermatologist takes a syringe with a tiny needle and places Artecoll into the wrinkle or furrow you want corrected. After injection, the doctor gently massages the Artecoll so it spreads and molds perfectly to fill the wrinkle, just like regular Collagen. Collagen implants alone do not last long, however. It is the microspheres in Artecoll that prevent wrinkles from reappearing. As the implanted collagen substance disappears, the microspheres implanted with it gradually blend with the rest of your tissue, so the wrinkle stays filled. You can think of Artecoll as a Collagen-like material that has found a way to last a lot longer.

Artecoll takes minutes to place into a wrinkle. An outpatient procedure, it is only slightly uncomfortable. As simple to perform as Collagen injections, it is especially used for wrinkles around the mouth, other deep wrinkles, frown lines, and lip enhancement. No anesthesia is necessary. Some side effects include temporary bruising and bleeding. A bumpiness to filled areas occasionally develops a few months following Artecoll implantation.

See also: Collagen, deep wrinkles, wrinkles

Astringents

Astringents help remove excess oil from skin, and are very helpful for those people with acne or oily skin. Astringents function the same way as toners, and the terms can be used interchangeably. These over-the-counter liquids are based on either witch hazel or alcohol in different strengths.

You can buy astringents almost anywhere. In general, if you buy them at salons and department stores they may cost more, but are often less irritating to the skin.

Astringents also help those with what is usually called "combination skin"—oily skin on the T-zone (central forehead, nose, and chin), and drier skin elsewhere on the face. Those people who have combination skin are usually advised to use the astringent exclusively in the T-zoned oily areas, and to moisturize the drier, outer parts of the face. Most dermatologists recommend the use of astringents on oily parts of the face not more than once or twice daily. Most dermatologists agree astringents should not be used on dry skin.

Autologen *[au-tol-o-jen]*

Autologen is a newer form of collagen injections. Unlike Collagen (derived from cows and trademarked) and Dermalogen (collagen derived from human tissue banks), Autologen comes from your own natural collagen. Biological collagen is a protein of the skin's undersurface that deteriorates over time, causing depressions in the skin, such as wrinkles.

Here's how the procedure works. Your dermatologist removes from your lower hip an inch-long, football-shaped piece of skin that is then sent to the makers of Autologen. They process the skin and send it back to the dermatologist in a syringe, ready for injection. The dermatologist is then able to fill scars and wrinkles with Autologen—your own skin's collagen.

(Alternatively, if you have a face-lift, the extra skin from the surgery can be sent to the makers of Autologen and made into injectable liquid collagen to fill in any wrinkles and lines at a later date.)

Injecting your own collagen virtually eliminates the risk of an allergic reaction. However, the procedure does leave a small scar on the hip.

This step of removing the piece of skin from your hip may one day be eliminated, as Autologen scientists hope to make Autologen using high-tech genetic engineering techniques. It is anticipated this new, improved Autologen will still have no risk of allergic reaction.

Autologen works best in the same places Collagen works—lines around the mouth and cheeks, and frown lines between the eyebrows. Like Collagen, Autologen treatment is not permanent, but it may last longer because it comes from you. Repeated treatments are still needed to maintain its effects, and treatment frequency depends upon your skin type and environmental factors.

See also: Collagen, Dermalogen, fat transplantation, Gore-Tex

Azelex *[az-a-lecks]* (azalaic acid)

Azelex or azalaic acid, a cream used for acne, has the side effect of lightening blotchy brown pigmentation or brown spots on the skin. It works like Retin-A in that it blocks the transfer of pigment granules from pigment cells to skin cells. It helps reduce pigmentation, but does not eliminate it.

Azalaic acid can be used with bleaching creams, Retin-A cream, the antiwrinkle cream Renova, kogic acid, or superficial chemical peels. In such combinations, azalaic acid becomes more effective in reducing blotchy brown pigmentation, skin discoloration (such as melasma), sun freckles, or brown pigmentation remaining after a rash.

See also: Bleaching cream, kogic acid, melasma, Renova, Retin-A, sun freckles, sunscreen

B

Baggy eyes

The natural process of age and gravity, with or without sun damage, slowly pulls on the soft skin beneath the eyes and over time loosens it into "bags." In addition, the loss of muscle tone over time sometimes causes the fat pads around the eyes to appear bigger.

Baggy eyes can be improved by blepharoplasty *[blef-ar-o-plas-tee]*, a surgery that removes the excess skin above and below the eyelids and the accompanying protruding fat pads. Some plastic surgeons perform this procedure by making an incision underneath the eyelid across the conjunctiva, the inside red margin part of the eye. This procedure is called a transconjunctival *[trans-con-junk-tie-val]* blepharoplasty.

Both types of blepharoplasty are done on an outpatient basis and take only a few hours. The result is tighter, more youthful-looking eyes. For more information, please see Eyelid Surgery on page 56.

Laser resurfacing of skin, a process often used to eliminate lines around the eyes, often referred to as "crow's feet," fails to help baggy eyes because it merely diminishes the wrinkles around the eyes without removing the bags and fat pads.

See also: CO_2 laser, eyelid surgery

Benign keratosis

Benign keratoses, also called seborrheic *[seb-or-ee-ik]* keratoses, are very common skin growths that are associated with the process of aging. They look like stuck-on brown or skin-colored spots that can be scaly or greasy. They can appear anywhere, including the face.

Medically, they present no health risk, but are often cosmetically undesirable. They do not disappear without medical intervention.

In a sense, they are an error in skin cell production. Benign keratosis occurs when, for no apparent reason, the skin produces identical clones of normal skin cells. The extra skin accumulates and forms these spots.

If you want to eliminate them, your dermatologist can remove them in several ways. One of the best and easiest ways is to freeze them; there may be a slight stinging pain. Other procedures include burning (or cauterizing), shaving, and scraping. In most cases, only very little scar tissue remains following their removal.

Beta glucan *[beta-glue-can]*

Beta glucan is a sugarlike compound derived from a yeast called saccharomyces. Beta glucan is thought to reduce sun damage, aid in antiaging, and speed the healing of wounds. This theory is based only on observations of beta glucan activity in laboratory petri dishes. We have no further evidence that beta glucan effectively reduces sun damage.

The Food and Drug Administration has not reviewed its usefulness as a skin-care remedy because there has never been a study done on humans. Nonetheless, beta glucan is available in some over-the-counter antiaging creams.

Betahydroxy *[beta-hie-drox-ee]* acids

Akin to alphahydroxy acids, betahydroxy acids are naturally derived compounds. True betahydroxy acids, like tropic acid, are not marketed as antiaging products. Instead, a compound called salicylic acid (that resembles a betahydroxy acid) is used to reduce wrinkles and sun-aged skin. Salicylic acid is often marketed as a betahydroxy acid because of their commonality, but technically they are not identical. Because the public and some practitioners use the acid terms interchangeably, this book lists salicylic as a betahydroxy acid for reference ease.

Salicylic acid has been used for decades as an effective antiacne medication. At present salicylic acid is also being used to help reduce the appearance of sun-damaged skin. Some dermatologists believe that salicylic acid, used in superficial peel strength formulation, can be as effective as but less irritating than alphahydroxy acids in reducing sun damage. Superficial peels of salicylic acid are being promoted to diminish brown blotching, iron out fine wrinkling, and tighten the skin for a smoother look.

Some dermatologists believe that salicylic acid in "lunchtime peel" strength may also be as effective as alphahydroxy acids in reducing skin discoloration, such as melasma. (Early reports seem to show that these peels may be safer than alphahydroxy acids in a broader range of skin pigmentation types.) Salicylic acid peels may be combined with over-the-counter or prescription-strength alphahydroxy acids or the antiwrinkle cream Renova to further reduce sun damage.

Low-concentration salicylic acid is available in some over-the-counter products; however, how those salicylic acid products compare with over-the-counter alphahydroxy acid creams is not known. These salicylic acid creams are sold as "betahydroxy acids," rather than as salicylic acid products.

See also: Alphahydroxy acids, chemical peels, melasma, photo damage, Renova, salicylic acid, small wrinkles, sun freckles, wrinkles

Bleaching cream

"Bleaching cream" is a generic term for topically applied cream that contains a chemical called hydroquinone *[hie-dro-kwin-own]*. Hydroquinones lighten skin because they retard pigment production through oxidization of the skin's pigment cells. Hydroquinones are the most widely prescribed medication sold in the United States for lightening skin discoloration. They are also available over the counter in lower strengths.

Hydroquinones are best used as part of a skin-lightening regimen. Applied alone, even prescription-strength hydroquinones do not usually work well enough to lighten spots significantly. Further, sun exposure often causes the lightened area to darken again. Consequently, dermatologists often use superficial chemical peels with either glycolic or salicylic acids that allow hydroquinones to better penetrate the skin and make them more effective.

Dermatologists also use Retin-A, the antiwrinkle cream Renova, and Azelex cream in combination with hydroquinones in order to bring about a more complete lightening that can blend seamlessly into the natural complexion of the skin. One prescription hydroquinone cream contains an added hint of glycolic acid to boost its efficacy.

With the help of a dermatologist, the right formula of hydroquinone can be found that will prevent possible skin irritation. Darkening, rather than lightening, of the skin can occur in darker-skinned people. Because of these risks, hydroquinones should be used in small amounts, and only under the care of a dermatologist.

See also: Alexandrite laser, alphahydroxy acids, Azelex, glycolic acid, kogic acid, lasers, melasma, Neodymium:Yag laser, salicylic acid, sun freckles

Blue Peel

Blue Peel was developed, trademarked, and marketed by Zein Obaji, M.D., a California dermatologist. This is a medium-depth chemical peel that uses a 30-percent trichloroacetic acid (TCA) solution and turns it into a somewhat safer paste, with a final concentration falling within the 15 to 20 percent range.

The Blue Peel lessens sun-damaged skin, wrinkles, unwanted brown spots, and superficial acne scars. Dr. Obaji added a blue hue to this peel in order to determine the consistency and uniformity of its effect on the skin. Therefore, your doctor can tell by the shade of blue how deep the peel has penetrated your skin. When penetration reaches the right depth, the face is then scrubbed with a green cleansing soap to remove the blue glow.

This peel is somewhat painful. You will probably want to take a light oral sedative before the procedure. Afterward, expect redness and peeling for several days to two weeks, depending on the strength of your peel.

A few side effects have been reported, including activation of herpes infection, severe scabbing, pigmentation irregularities, and scarring. The use of the antiwrinkle cream Renova for several weeks prior to a Blue Peel will enhance its effectiveness.

See also: Chemical peels

Botox (botulism toxin)

Botox is an abbreviated term for botulism toxin, derived from botulism bacteria, a dreaded chemical commonly known to cause food poisoning. When used as part of a skin-care regimen, however, Botox can create younger-looking skin.

In creating Botox, scientists dilute the botulism toxin for medical purposes. The FDA has approved its use for treatment of eye muscle spasms or involuntary neck muscle twitches. However, eye doctors, dermatologists, plastic surgeons, and even neurologists have since learned that the muscle-weakening powers of Botox can have cosmetic applications as well.

When Botox is injected through a small needle into the middle of a muscle, it can cause temporary weakening of that muscle. How does this make people look younger? Such an application is useful for people who want to lessen the thick furrows in their foreheads, or "frown" lines between their eyes and in the immediate area above their eyes. When Botox is injected into the muscles that control these folds, the muscles relax, and the furrowed lines created by muscle tension slacken and vanish. The creation of smoother, softer-looking skin is the most popular cosmetic application of Botox.

Less commonly, people who have very prominent muscles around the "crow's feet" around their eyes or thick prominent muscles in the center of the neck can have these overused muscles relaxed through an injection of Botox. In fact, some dermatologists use Botox to relax neck muscles and create a mini (lower) face- and neck-lift in people who cannot undergo surgical face-lifts.

If you have Botox placed into your forehead muscles, you risk having droopy eyelids or fallen eyebrows for up to several weeks after injection. While this risk can be minimized by following the very specific aftercare guidelines provided by your doctor, on rare occasions they still do occur. The wrinkle-relaxing effects of Botox are not permanent, and repeat injections are needed to maintain wrinkle relaxation. *See also:* Deep wrinkles, Collagen

Breast implants

Many women undergo breast implant surgery, also known as breast augmentation or augmentation mammoplasty, to make their breasts firmer and more youthful looking. Breast augmentation is not a substitute for a breast lift, a procedure used to raise sagging breasts and make them firmer. Plastic surgeons can perform breast augmentation in their offices or at a local hospital's outpatient surgical center. The surgery usually takes less than two hours and either general anesthesia, or local anesthesia and a sedative, is used.

Once you are sedated or anesthetized, your plastic surgeon selects one of three small incisions to place the implants into your breasts. These incisions are usually made underneath the breast, armpit, or nipple. All of the incision lines are engineered to hide any subsequent scars. After creating some space in your breast tissue, your surgeon can place the implants either under the breast tissue or even further under the muscle in the chest. Although initially more painful, implants placed under the muscle may interfere less with future mammograms and the standard examination for abnormal breast conditions.

After breast augmentation surgery, you may have some tenderness around your breasts or a burning sensation around your nipples. Your breasts may also be somewhat bruised for a few weeks.

A saline-filled implant is most often used today. Saline is a salty fluid that is naturally found in the body. In the unlikely event the implant ruptures, the saline solution is safely absorbed by the body. The FDA has approved this implant. Other implant substances are not currently FDA approved.

Uncommon side effects from breast augmentation surgery include a tight scar or infection around the implant, and a decrease or increase in sensation around the nipples. To obtain the best results you should follow your plastic surgeon's guidelines before and after surgery.
See also: Breast lift

Breast lift

For many women, age, gravity, pregnancy, and breast-feeding contribute to loose and sagging breasts. A breast lift, also known as mastoplexy, is an outpatient procedure many women undergo to regain the firm breasts they may have lost due to one or more of these factors. Performed by plastic surgeons, mastoplexy reshapes your breasts so that they are higher and firmer. Unlike breast augmentation, mastoplexy does not increase the size of your breasts. However, breast lift surgery can be performed in conjunction with breast augmentation.

The process is as follows: Under general anesthesia, your surgeon basically removes excess skin and places your nipples higher up on your breasts. Incisions are usually made around your nipple and the contours of your breasts. Mastoplexy is usually completed in less than three hours. Breast lift surgery is usually performed in your plastic surgeon's office or in an outpatient surgical center at your local hospital. Occasionally, people may stay in the hospital for a day or two.

After the surgery, your breasts may be bruised, tender, and swollen. It is important to follow your plastic surgeon's aftercare instructions carefully. Although it is rare, infection, bleeding, or loss of sensation around the nipples can occur. The benefits of breast lift surgery are not permanent and you can expect that the effects of gravity will eventually cause your breasts to sag again in the future.

Buf-Puf

First introduced about twenty-five years ago, the Buf-Puf is a sponge engineered to exfoliate the skin. Sold over the counter, the sponge is comprised of polyester fibers, and comes in three different textures. People who have more sensitive skin are advised to start with the extra gentle texture, while those who have tougher skin can start with the regular texture. The superiority of the Buf-Puf to other exfoliating procedures, such as over-the-counter glycolic and salicylic acids or facials, has not been proven in scientific studies. When used as part of a daily skin-care regimen, however, results, such as smoother skin and texture, can occur.

C

CO$_2$ laser (carbon dioxide laser)

The CO$_2$, or carbon dioxide, laser has been used by medical professionals for almost two decades. The carbon dioxide laser, unlike newer lasers that target a specific color (such as red in blood vessels or brown in pigmented spots), vaporizes and chars anything with water content. Since all skin contains water, it destroys every bit of skin or tissue it contacts. Without local anesthesia or sedation, treatments using the CO$_2$ laser are extremely painful.

Until recently, the CO$_2$ laser was used primarily for destroying warts, eliminating small benign growths, and smoothing out growths such as "W. C. Field's nose," as seen in patients with an advanced skin condition called rosacea. It was also used in lieu of a scalpel in patients who take blood thinners because blood coagulates immediately after the skin is cut with this laser. The high degree of charring that occurs with the CO$_2$ laser, however, limits its usefulness for medical procedures, especially those that require a positive cosmetic outcome.

During the past decade, however, the use of the CO$_2$ laser has mushroomed because of the development of "superpulsed" CO$_2$ lasers. The superpulsed laser has high-frequency, microsecond pulses that allow for precision performance. Superpulsed lasers can vaporize microscopic layers of skin cells so that the depth of penetration and hence the risks of scarring or poor cosmetic outcome can be significantly lowered. The superpulsed CO$_2$ lasers are commonly used to restore a more youthful look by resurfacing or dermabrading sun-damaged and wrinkled skin. It is possible to have an entire face resurfaced or just the areas around the eyes or mouth. The lasers can also be used to smooth out deep acne scars. A medical benefit of this laser is to destroy multiple precancerous growths, called solar keratoses.

Although the depth of penetration is controlled, these lasers still abrade deep enough to cause at least the entire top layer of skin to be removed. Thus, patients who undergo a procedure with the superpulsed CO_2 lasers have a significantly longer recovery period (several weeks to several months) than those who undergo superficial and medium-depth chemical peels (up to ten days). In terms of depth of penetration and recovery time, the CO_2 laser is comparable to a deep chemical peel, such as a phenol peel.

During the recovery period, a person's face is very raw looking and may be scabbed, because the sun-damaged skin has been removed, and the new skin needs time to regenerate. After the skin heals, some individuals may have blotchy brown pigmentation, persistent redness, and in rare instances, scarring. Most scientists believe that lighter-skinned people obtain more favorable outcomes with fewer side effects than darker-skinned people. This CO_2 resurfaced skin does not always stay smooth permanently, and sun-damaged skin may likely recur after several years. Most dermatologists believe that this laser should be reserved for individuals who have a large degree of sun damage and deep wrinkles and who do not mind making a greater commitment to after-laser care and recovery time. Using the anti-wrinkle cream Renova for several weeks prior to laser resurfacing may enhance its effectiveness.

See also: Deep wrinkles, dermabrasion, Erbium:Yag laser, phenol peels, photo damage

Camouflage

Camouflaging implies covering up unwanted spots and irregularities through the use of different kinds of makeup, particularly foundation. Foundations come in different textures, such as liquid, cream, stick, and cake form. Usually lighter-skinned people need only blend a maximum of eight colors to achieve a cover-up, while darker-skinned people may need up to thirty-five colors to conceal a deep scar, blemish, or unwanted age spot.

The best camouflage creams are the heavier makeup products because they provide better coverage than the watery lotions. The disadvantage to these camouflage creams is that they may feel heavy, and are more likely to aggravate acne-prone or oily skin. For oily skin choose a foundation that has low or no oil content; for dry skin opt for a moisture-based foundation. Foundation should be applied from the top of your face toward the bottom with a downward stroke. To even out skin color irregularities, apply a small amount of foundation at the jawline to ensure the color is harmonious and blends with the natural tones of the face and neck. No lines of demarcation should be seen. Darker shaded foundations help to blend elevated areas, while lighter-shaded foundations are used to cover depressed areas.

Cautery *[kot-er-ee]*

Cauterization is a technique that dermatologists have been using for decades. A very fine electric needle is used that chars and hence destroys anything it touches. It is generally used to eliminate small benign growths such as benign keratoses, tiny red growths called cherry angiomas, and spider veins on the face. Spider veins on the legs and elsewhere on the body do not respond to cautery; lasers or sclerotherapy are used to eliminate veins in these locations.

Cauterization at a low setting is somewhat uncomfortable, but can usually be performed without the use of local anesthesia. If the growth is deep, local anesthesia is necessary.
See also: Benign keratosis, spider veins

Celex-C *[sel-x-see]*

An over-the-counter product that is sold at salons, department stores, and dermatologist's offices, Celex-C is probably the most commercially available form of topical vitamin C. Vitamin C helps destroy free radicals, the toxic molecules that are formed from sun exposure and cause damage to the skin. Unfortunately, the skin does not easily absorb topically applied vitamin C.

Both Celex-C and other vitamin C cream manufacturers believe that their formulas facilitate vitamin C penetration. Research studies have documented that topically applied vitamin C provides sunscreen-like effectiveness in protecting the skin against the rays of the sun. Thus, when used in conjunction with sunscreens, Celex-C and other similar vitamin C products appear to help protect the skin from sun damage and prevent skin cancer. Some researchers also believe that Celex-C and related vitamin C products restore a youthful glow to the skin and remove facial wrinkles and other aspects of sun-damaged skin. However, this particular claim has yet to be supported by clinical tests.

For more information on products like Celex-C, please see Vitamin C on page 124.

See also: Free radicals, photo damage, sun damage, sun protection, sunscreen, vitamin C

Cellulite

Cellulite is a medical term for fat, specifically lumpy fat located around the upper thighs and lower buttocks. Cellulite affects many more women than men: It is estimated that almost 85 percent of American women have excessive cellulite on their thighs and buttocks.

How do our bodies create cellulite? The latest theory suggests that female hormonal influences cause fat cells to cluster together in the thighs. The clumped fat cells constrict the tiny local blood vessels and impair normal blood flow. With damaged blood vessels and compromised blood flow, the cells in the thigh area cannot repair themselves in their usual way. Instead, deposits of protein form around the clumped fat cells and damaged blood vessels. The combination of protein and fat with poor circulation creates spots under the skin, which project a "cottage cheese" appearance in the thighs. In short, scientists now think cellulite is a consequence of female hormones, decreased circulation in tiny blood vessels, and protein and fat globule deposits under the skin. Much of this process may be genetically determined.

Over-the-counter creams for the thighs contain one or more ingredients that are reported to destroy fat deposits, and thereby deter the formation of cellulite. Research studies have shown at best only minimal improvement with creams that contain caffeine. Cream-based products with botanical ingredients, such as sweet clover, ivy barley, lemon, kola nut, fennel, algae, and strawberry, are also advertised for cellulite. To date, nobody knows how these substances affect cellulite, and no well-designed research studies support the claims of these over-the-counter creams. Massaging the thighs to promote good circulation is another technique used to reduce cellulite. Many spas use a combination of herbs and other naturally derived creams, in conjunction with massage, heating pads, or warm towels. A special machine called Endermologie is also used to help massage the skin and promote circulation. Endermologie experts claim their machine increases local circulation as the clusters of cellulite are rolled over and stretched out. Endermologie machines are used by some dermatologists and plastic surgeons, and may temporarily reduce cellulite when combined with a healthy diet and regular exercise program. A healthy diet and a regular exercise program appear to control cellulite by stimulating circulation and metabolism.

Liposuction is a surgical procedure used to reduce cellulite. After an incision, a small metal tube is placed in the fat site, and a pumplike device suctions unwanted fat from the body. Scientific literature suggests that this is the most effective way to achieve visible results. Liposuction, however, involves a certain amount of risk and should be discussed with your dermatologist or plastic surgeon. Liposuction acts only to reduce fatty deposits; it does not address the problems of circulation or hormone influence that contribute to cellulite. Although liposuction appears to provide the most visible results, future treatments that target fat removal as well as circulation and hormone influences would remove cellulite even more effectively.

See also: Fat removal, liposuction, thigh creams

Cheek implants (or Malar augmentation)

Genetic as well as environmental factors contribute to sunken cheeks. If you think your cheeks have become "depressed" with age, adding implants will add definition to your face and provide a more youthful appearance. Cheek implants are generally performed by facial plastic surgeons who use a local anesthetic to numb the cheeks. Recovery time is usually confined to one week.

Cheeks can be filled with both natural and synthetic substances. Body fat, often taken from the hip, is removed with a syringe, and put through a special process before it is placed in the cheeks. However, fat placed this way does dissolve with time, which means that periodic touch-ups are needed. Synthetic materials such as Gore-Tex are popular because Gore-Tex can be molded more easily to provide a particular look. The procedure is reversible when synthetic materials are used, so if you are not pleased with the result the implant can be further manipulated. In addition, Gore-Tex lasts a lot longer, perhaps indefinitely, compared to natural fillers, so touch-ups are not needed.

See also: Face-lift, fat removal, Gore-Tex

Chemical peels (superficial, medium, deep)

Chemical peels come in many different varieties. They are best classified by the degree to which they penetrate the skin. Depth of skin penetration determines the extent to which the skin can be rejuvenated. During this procedure a chemical is wiped on the skin, left on for a specified length of time, and then removed.

Superficial chemical peels come in either salon or prescription strength, both referred to as "lunchtime peels" because they are virtually free of side effects and the person can return to work within the hour without anyone there knowing that the procedure was done. The term "peel" is really a misnomer, because not much peeling occurs. These peels cause an improvement in the skin that lasts from several weeks to months and need to be repeated to maintain their effect. The results are enhanced when they are used with a daily home regimen of alphahydroxy acids and/or the antiwrinkle cream Renova.

Salon-strength superficial peels are usually made from a low concentration of glycolic acid (an alphahydroxy acid), and are performed by staffs in salons and other spas. These superficial peels gently exfoliate the skin, giving it a temporary, but refreshing healthy glow. Salon peels are probably insufficient to restore sun-damaged skin or to fade brown spots.

Prescription-strength superficial peels are made from varying concentrations of glycolic acid (usually 30 to 70 percent free—or available—acid), 20 to 30 percent salicylic acid, 10 percent trichloracetic acid (TCA), and an agent called Jessner's solution. This type of peel is performed in a dermatologist's or plastic surgeon's office. The procedure gives the skin a healthy glow, and when repeated, reverses some of the features of sun-damaged skin. These peels can also help lessen irregular blotchiness and unwanted brown spots such as melasma. Their effect on reversing sun damage and unwanted brown spots is enhanced with the use of daily bleaching creams, Azelex cream, or Retin-A. No sedation or local anesthesia is necessary for superficial chemical peels, as they are, at most, only slightly uncomfortable.

Superficial "lunchtime" peels are generally safest for lighter-skinned people, but some dermatologists think that they can be safely used on all skin colors. Salicylic acid peels are somewhat safer than other superficial peels for darker-skinned individuals. The main risk of these peels is the possibility of irregular pigmentation. The procedure occasionally causes facial redness and peeling for several days. Fortunately, these side effects are uncommon, but if they occur you should notify your dermatologist immediately.

Medium-depth chemical peels can be performed with higher concentrations of TCA (20 to 40 percent), or by combining lower strengths of TCA with Jessner's peel or high-strength glycolic acids. (Many dermatologists prefer medium-depth peels in a paste rather than liquid form, because pastes tend to give more consistent results.) By definition, all medium-depth peels are deeper, more effective, and have a longer-lasting outcome than superficial chemical peels. One peel generally lasts for up to a year. They are usually reserved for people who want to improve moderate to severe sun damage, or (less commonly) to remove unwanted pigmentation and precancerous growths called solar keratoses. Because medium-depth peels can be quite uncomfortable, an oral sedative is often prescribed prior to the procedure. Peeling can last from several days to two weeks, so these individuals may want to take a few days off from work after such a procedure. Because excessive peeling or skin erosions may occur, you need to follow the aftercare instructions of your dermatologist or plastic surgeon. Medium-depth chemical peels are typically enhanced by using the antiwrinkle cream Renova for several weeks beforehand.

Risks include severe peeling, increased irregular pigmentation, activation of herpes infection on the face, and scarring. These risks are uncommon.

Deep chemical peels are comparable in strength to laser skin resurfacing, and are usually performed with a chemical called phenol. As with laser resurfacing, they are best reserved for people who want to reverse the effects of severe sun damage and wrinkles. Phenol peels, like the superpulsed CO_2 laser, also help reduce acne scarring and unwanted brown spots. The result of a phenol peel is very long lasting and usually does not need to be repeated. Unlike lasers, phenol peels have been performed by dermatologists and plastic surgeons for over thirty years and thus have a very good track record.

Because the pain from a phenol peel is similar to the pain from CO_2 laser resurfacing, intravenous sedatives or anesthesia is used. After applying the phenol peel, petrolatum is usually applied to the skin for forty-eight hours. These peels rarely cause permanent heart damage, but heart monitoring is essential during the procedure. Intravenous fluids are also given to help reduce the risk of kidney damage. Phenol peels are usually performed in several segments taking from sixty to ninety minutes to complete. One can expect severe redness, peeling, and sometimes scabbing after a phenol peel. At least several weeks may pass before the results of younger, healthy-looking skin are seen. Obviously, it is necessary to follow very specific physician instructions in order to reduce unwanted risks, which can include increased blotchiness, long-lasting redness, and scarring.

Used primarily to decrease the appearance of wrinkles, sun spots, and blotchiness, and to enhance an overall healthy glow to the skin, chemical peels are not substitutes for face-lifts and do not repair sagging skin.

See also: Blue peel, CO_2 laser, deep wrinkles, glycolic acid, phenol peel, photo damage, Renova, salicylic acid, TCA

Chin implants

Because the chin may have receded with time, chin implants restore its prominence, thereby making the entire face appear more sturdy and youthful. Often, chin implants are needed after a nose job, or rhinoplasty *[rye-no-plas-tee]*, in order to even out the face and make the chin aesthetically compatible with the nose. Chin implants are also often performed after liposuction under the chin to even out the facial profile. Chin implants are usually performed by plastic surgeons, only occasionally by dermatologists.

Several filling substances are now available to fill the chin area, such as Silastic *[sie-las-tik]* Gore-Tex or fat. Fat can be removed from your hip with a syringe, and prepared by the physician so that it can be injected into your chin. You can't have an allergic reaction to your own fat. On the other hand, because the fat transplanted into the chin is eventually absorbed, the result doesn't last long, unless the procedure is repeated occasionally. In contrast, Silastic and Gore-Tex are synthetic, permanent materials that should last a lifetime. Silastic is sturdy, but bendable plastic-like material that is inserted through a small incision site in the middle of your chin, and then fitted into your chin by covering it from one side of your jawbone to the other. Gore-Tex comes in somewhat more flexible sheets or blocks that can be placed into a small incision in your chin with a special instrument.

The chin area is numbed with local anesthesia, and the outpatient procedure is normally completed in less than an hour. Sometimes intravenous or oral sedatives are used. Side effects include temporary bruising, swelling, and tenderness. *See also:* Alloderm, fat transplantation, Gore-Tex

Collagen *[kol-a-jen]*
Collagen is a fibrous-like material in the skin that helps give it strength. As we age, and especially as we expose ourselves to sun, collagen fibers become disorganized and decrease in number and strength. Because sun-damaged skin lacks the ability to reorganize and produce new collagen, wrinkles appear.

About two decades ago, a company in Northern California trademarked a form of collagen purified from cow skin to correct wrinkles. This Collagen is a thick white liquid that is implanted by dermatologists with a very fine needle directly into the wrinkles that need correction. Even though it is purified from cow skin, in most instances human skin accepts this injection with few side effects. Smaller wrinkles around the mouth and cheeks are usually injected with a thinner version of Collagen, while deeper wrinkles are injected with a thicker version.

Usually, people elect to have Collagen injections to achieve fuller lips or to have frown lines and lines around the mouth reduced or eliminated. Collagen implanted by this method usually lasts anywhere from several months to a few years before being absorbed by the body. Once this occurs, the skin returns to its prior condition. Repeat Collagen treatments are therefore necessary. Because Collagen is made from cows and not human skin, prior to treatment two test implants in the skin on the arm (separated by at least two weeks) are necessary to determine whether there is an allergic response to it.

Possible side effects of Collagen treatments include some bruising and redness at the injected sites for several days. A rare complication is the formation of a large, red, swollen growth at the injection site.

For most of the past two decades, Collagen has been the only injectable collagen available to correct sun-induced wrinkling. Autologen, or collagen derived from one's own skin, has recently become available. Other filling substances for deeper wrinkles, such as Dermalogen, are now also available and compete with Collagen. A dermatologist can help you decide the best treatment for your skin type.

See also: Autologen, Dermalogen, fat transplantation, Isolagen

Color wheel

The color wheel is the guide aestheticians and makeup specialists use to cover up unwanted spots and blemishes and blend them with the skin's natural color. A circular diagram of the color spectrum, the color wheel is made of pie slices of green, blue, purple, red, orange, and yellow. You select the color on the wheel opposite the one you want to conceal, and apply a camouflage makeup of that opposite color. Instantaneously and perfectly, you have just camouflaged the spot you wanted to hide through the use of colors on the color wheel.

For example, if you are left after laser surgery with a purple bruise, applying a yellow-based makeup will conceal the bruise and leave the skin looking close to its normal color. (This is because the color opposite purple on the color wheel is yellow.)

D

Dark circles under the eyes

Dark circles usually occur as we get older, although some people appear more prone to them than others. They are not the result of sun exposure or an effect from tanning. Scientists do not know what causes these.

However, there are a few treatments dermatologists use to decrease these dark circles; unfortunately, none of these therapies provides the perfect answer. One treatment you may want to try is kogic acid, a brown spot-removing gel. It can be purchased from a dermatologist and is simple to apply. Because kogic acid can be irritating and potentially cause these circles to become darker, you must follow your doctor's specific instructions. Kogic acid takes a few months before a result is seen.

Bleaching creams are another way dark circles can be lightened. Unfortunately, these creams are not usually very effective. Some dermatologists also use vitamin K creams with or without bleaching creams to lighten dark circles under the eyes. Lasers are the newest method used to reduce the prominence of dark circles. In a few small studies, the Alexandrite and Neodymium:Yag lasers were found to reduce dark circles under the eyes significantly. Side effects include temporary bruising and swelling around the eyes.

See also: Alexandrite laser, bleaching creams, Kogic acid, Neodymium:Yag laser

Deep wrinkles

Deep wrinkles are the result of sun damage. In sun-damaged, or photo-aged skin, the natural collagen is an abnormal "elastic-like" material; we see this as a crevice, or a deep wrinkle.

The best way to combat deep wrinkles is to protect yourself from the damaging rays of the sun. Sunscreen applied appropriately, the use of hats and scarves to shield your face, and avoidance of the peak hours of 10:00 a.m. to 3:00 p.m. are basic prevention measures. As smoking contributes to deep wrinkles around the mouth, this habit is best avoided.

Once a deep wrinkle has formed, there are a number of options: you can fill the wrinkle, relax the wrinkle, or remove the wrinkle. Collagen, Autologen, Gore-Tex, Botox, fat transplantation, laser resurfacing, and dermabrasion are just some available options. A dermatologist can help to select the most appropriate treatment.

See also: Autologen, Botox, Collagen, dermabrasion, Dermalogen, fat transplantation, Gore-Tex, laser resurfacing, SoftForm, Sunscreen

Dermabrasion

A dermabrasion removes the top layers of skin so that newer, smoother skin can replace them. Usually people undergo dermabrasion to get rid of sun-damaged skin; when new skin grows to replace it, the face looks healthier and younger. Dermabrasion is not meant to remove excess, or baggy facial skin, nor is it a substitute for a face-lift.

The classic technique dermatologists have used for many years employs a sterilized electric sanding device. When this electric "sander" is applied to the skin, it removes the skin layer by layer. The depth of dermabrasion is determined by the number of layers that are removed.

One of the challenges of classic dermabrasion is the even removal of the same amount of skin from all areas of the face. Bleeding during this procedure may further detract from your doctor's visual field. A good dermabrasion only removes enough layers to allow new skin to grow back and provide a younger, fresher look.

After dermabrasion, the face is very red and raw-looking. It may take many months to heal, but the healing process can be accelerated by carefully following your physician's aftercare instructions. Most people elect not to go out in public for several weeks after the procedure. Dermabrasion appears to work best for lighter-skinned people.

Once healed, however, prior fine and deep wrinkling, acne scars, and blotchy, brown pigmentation are no longer on the face. A dermabrasion lasts for at least several years, if not longer.

Because dermabrasion can be quite painful, intravenous sedation is required. Some dermatologists perform localized dermabrasions in order to smooth out raised or depressed scars, or post-surgical scars. This is done with the same sterile electric sanding machine used in a facial dermabrasion, but for a shorter period of time. Sometimes a dermatologist may simply use a special sandpaper-type material and hand sand the raised skin imperfection in order to even it out with the rest of the skin. With small areas of dermabrasion a localized anesthetic is injected. This process takes only a few weeks to heal.

In the past decade, dermabrasion has been changed by the use of lasers such as the superpulsed CO_2 and Erbium:Yag lasers. These remove the top layers of the skin so it can regrow with a healthier, smoother look. However, laser dermabrasion is much easier to control, much easier to gauge, and is practically bloodless compared to classic dermabrasion.

Laser dermabrasion is also called laser resurfacing. The superpulsed CO_2 and Erbium:Yag lasers have high-frequency, microsecond pulses that allow for precision performance. The lasers vaporize microscopic layers of skin cells so that the depth of penetration—and hence risks including scarring—can be closely controlled. You can elect to have your entire face resurfaced or just the areas around the eyes or mouth. Lasers can also be used to smooth out deep acne scars. In general, laser dermabrasion is preferred over classic methods.

The Erbium:Yag laser gives a more superficial dermabrasion than the superpulsed CO_2 laser. Not as much sun-damaged skin is removed, and the recovery period is shorter. Still, the recovery period from the Erbium:Yag laser is one or two weeks longer than the recovery period following superficial chemical peels (which is negligible).

The superpulsed CO_2 laser is comparable to a deep chemical peel, such as a phenol peel, in terms of depth of penetration and recovery time. Because this procedure is painful it requires intravenous sedation. During the recovery period, the face is very raw-looking and may be scabbed, because the sun-damaged skin has been removed, and the new skin needs time to grow and regenerate. After the skin heals, blotchy brown pigmentation, persistent redness, and in rare instances, scarring, sometime occurs. Many scientists believe that lighter-skinned people tolerate and heal more safely after laser resurfacing than darker-skinned people. The effects of laser dermabrasion are also not always permanent, and sun-damaged skin can recur after several years.

See also: Chemical peels, CO_2 laser, deep wrinkles, Erbium:Yag laser, lasers, photo damage

Dermalogen

One way to fill deep crevices and wrinkles is with Dermalogen, a new high-tech product from the researchers who developed the wrinkle-filler Autologen. Dermalogen is a liquid injectable material that dermatologists can place directly into unwanted wrinkles. Dermalogen is made by taking tissue from a human skin bank and purifying it into an injectable human collagen, a skin protein. In a way, it is similar to Alloderm, another skin bank product purified into a collagen substance, except Alloderm is produced as a semi-solid material to implant into deeper crevices, while Dermalogen is an injectable liquid.

Dermalogen and the brand-name product Collagen are both injectable collagen products used to reduce the signs of wrinkles; however, Dermalogen is derived from collagen from human skin, whereas Collagen mainly consists of puri-fied collagen in cow's skin. Because it is derived from human beings, Dermalogen is less likely than Collagen to produce an allergic response. It may last longer as well, but you will still require occasional repeat injections to maintain wrinkle-free skin.

The lines between the eyebrows on the forehead (frown lines), and around the mouth seem to respond best to Dermalogen injections. No anesthesia is necessary, although some minor discomfort may accompany the injections. The main side effects of Dermalogen are temporary bruising and minor redness at the injection sites.

See also: Artecoll, Autologen, Collagen, deep wrinkles, Isolagen

Desiccation *[dess-a-kae-shun]*

Desiccation is another term for cautery, a technique that dermatologists have been using for decades. A very fine electric needle is used that chars and therefore destroys anything it touches. Desiccation at a low setting is somewhat uncomfortable, but the procedure can usually be performed without the use of local anesthesia. If a growth is deep, local anesthesia is often necessary. Dermatologists use the method to remove small benign growths on the face, such as benign keratoses, small red growths called cherry angiomas, and spider veins. Because spider veins on the legs and elsewhere on the body do not respond to desiccation, lasers or sclerotherapy are used there.

See also: benign keratosis, spider veins

DHEA (dihydroepiandosterone)

DHEA (dihydroepiandosterone *[die-hie-dro-epee-an-dos-terown]*) pills are one of the most popular items sold in health food stores today. Many people believe that taking this male hormone in pill form will help them look and feel younger. Unfortunately, DHEA's usefulness as a "fountain of youth" has not been proved and the health risks of taking it on a daily basis are unknown. Interestingly, DHEA applied topically in cream form may be an effective skin moisturizer. Before you try DHEA, discuss its benefits and potential side effects with your doctor.

See also: Hormone creams

Diet

A healthy diet is always good for the mind and body. Eating a vitamin-rich, well-balanced diet is unquestionably helpful for every organ in the body, including the skin. Low-fat and low-cholesterol diets can help prevent heart disease. Adequate daily fiber intake helps keep the gastrointestinal tract regular and unconstipated. Vitamins C and E are antioxidants that when taken in foods or as supplements may diminish the risk of sunburn.

On the other hand, some widely accepted notions about diet and skin have yet to be proven. For example, although many people can trace acne directly to their ingesting greasy foods or chocolate, to date scientists have not found evidence to support this claim. Drinking six 6-ounce glasses of water on a daily basis (as generally advised) is not as effective as applying moisturizers on a regular basis.

Inadequate food intake leading to vitamin and nutrient deficiencies does affect the skin's appearance adversely. Crash dieting, anorexia nervosa, or rapid weight loss can contribute to hair loss and brittle nails. Excessive intake of carrots and beta-carotene, a form of vitamin A, can result in an orange discoloration of the skin. It seems that too much or too little of anything we eat has the potential to disturb the delicate balance of well-being. For optimum health, most doctors recommend a well-balanced diet, a regular exercise program, and vitamin supplementation taken under their supervision.

See also: Nutrition, vitamin A, vitamin C, vitamin E

Diode laser

Since diode lasers are a recent development in laser technology, not much information is available on them. The diode device makes these lasers both powerful and versatile, yet they are very small machines. Dermatologists find them to be much more reliable and maintenance-free than other types of lasers. Dermatologists are just starting to use them for hair and spider vein removal. In the future probably they will be used for other skin applications.

See also: Hair removal, lasers

Dry skin

As people age their skin often becomes drier. At first, we may find our hands and feet are dry; later, the arms and legs are affected. Because the face has the greatest number of oil glands (which preserve moisture in the skin), it is usually the last skin surface to become dry.

Sun exposure contributes to dry skin. Sun-aged, or photo-aged, skin is rougher and more weathered than skin that has not been exposed to sun rays. Skin also becomes drier in the winter, when the air becomes drier and colder. Dry heat from home furnaces in winter further contributes to dry skin conditions.

Frequent moisturizing with the proper kinds of creams and moisturizers help control and replenish dry skin. In general, lighter moisturizers called lotions are fine to use on mildly dry skin, but moderate to severely dry skin requires heavier cream-based moisturizers. Bathing in products that contain such soothing ingredients as oatmeal may relieve some itchiness related to dry skin.

Doctors also recommend a diet rich in omega-3 fatty acids, and the oral or topical use of vitamins, such as vitamin E creams. Increasing your daily water intake will help, but is not as effective as topical cream or oil application.

See also: Moisturizers, photo damage

E

Electrolysis

Electrolysis, one of the most popular methods of hair removal, is a procedure performed by licensed professionals called electrologists. Hair is removed *permanently*, as opposed to temporary methods of hair removal like shaving, waxing, and epilation. An electric current (with or without high heat) destroys each hair down to its roots. Most commonly, a blend of heat and electric current is used.

Although results are excellent, electrolysis is a painful and time-consuming process. The electrologist first needs to find the root of each hair follicle with a magnifying glass before burning it. Often, only twenty-five to seventy-five hairs can be treated in one visit. Multiple visits to the electrologist's office are therefore necessary in order to complete hair removal in one area. Preferred areas of treatment are bikini lines, underarms, eyebrows, and chin and upper lip areas. In order to relieve some, but not all, of the pain from electrolysis, electrologists often have dermatologists prescribe topical anesthetic creams for their clients to apply just prior to treatment.

Sometimes dermatologists and electrologists work directly together. The dermatologist injects an anesthetic into the area treated. Then the electrologist painlessly removes hair from the numbed area. After a number of treatments, the vast majority of hairs removed with electrolysis are permanently eliminated. However, there is a small percentage of hairs that can regrow. Laser hair removal is now the chief competition for electrolysis because it can cover large areas more quickly.

See also: Lasers, waxing

Erbium:Yag laser

The Erbium:Yag laser (named from its use of the elements erbium, yttrium, aluminum, and garnet) is primarily used for the removal of light facial wrinkles. The combination of elements allows the laser to emit light energy at its unique water-absorbing wavelength, which is invisible to the human eye. The procedure is usually done in the dermatologist's or plastic surgeon's office. When the Erbium:Yag laser is used to remove wrinkles just around the eyes or mouth, local anesthesia is enough. When used on the entire face, oral or intravenous sedation is often used.

Removing wrinkles is generally done through a process called dermabrasion, and the laser most commonly used for this is the advanced superpulsed CO_2 laser. The Erbium: Yag laser is a newer instrument used for the same purpose. However, the superpulsed CO_2 laser penetrates deeper than the Erbium:Yag laser. Thus, the CO_2 laser can remove deeper wrinkles than the Erbium:Yag laser. If you have wrinkles that are not very deep, and want to add a fresher healthier glow to your face, the Erbium:Yag laser may be the treatment of choice.

While you are healing, some swelling, redness, and scabbing may occur. After either laser treatment, it is usually necessary to take a short leave of absence from work. Healing after a laser dermabrasion with the Erbium:Yag laser takes at most a few weeks, whereas recuperation after the CO_2 laser dermabrasion can take several months. Your doctor can help you decide which laser procedure is best for you.

See also: CO_2 laser, dermabrasion

Ethocyn *[eth-o-sin]*

Ethocyn is a topically applied cream that may block the production of male hormones in the skin. Since male hormones can suppress production of elastin, an elastic tissue protein in unwrinkled skin, it is believed that after daily application of Ethocyn, the skin will increase its production of elastin, and therefore decrease the formation of wrinkles.

Some studies done with Ethocyn show an increase in elastin-like material after two months of use. Because these Ethocyn studies have not been authenticated, the theory in not accepted by most dermatologists. Available since 1994, Ethocyn is an over-the-counter product sold in some salons and dermatologist offices.

Excessive hair

Cultural attitudes determine whether excessive hair growth on certain areas of the body is considered unappealing. For example, in many European countries, it is acceptable for women to have hair under their arms and on their legs, but in the United States, most women and men find it undesirable. Most American women would prefer to have little or no hair in places such as the abdomen, breasts, and face, specifically on the chin, upper lip, jawline, and between the eyebrows. Some men find excessive hair across their backs and shoulders unattractive.

Of the many methods available to remove excessive hair, electrolysis and depilatories are most popular. Electrolysis uses a blend of heat and electric current to remove hair. Electrolysis removes most hair permanently, but the process is slow. Depilatories are chemicals applied to the skin that loosen hair so it can be wiped away, although it eventually regrows.

The removal of hair by waxing is usually done in a salon or a spa. Waxing appears to be preferred more by women than by men. Both hot waxes and cold waxes are now available, and are especially popular for the removal of hair on the chin, eyebrow, and groin. Waxing can be painful, and may burn the skin, sometimes so severely a visit to the dermatologist is required. Another slight risk is infection of the hair follicles from which hairs have been removed. Hairs removed by waxing do grow back, but much more slowly than shaved hair.

Lasers are much less painful than all of the above procedures and significantly faster. Laser hair removal is performed by dermatologists and plastic surgeons. They work by targeting the pigment cells that are located on each hair beneath the skin. It often takes only one treatment to remove the unwanted hair. At present, lasers' ability to remove excessive hair permanently is the same as electrolysis, but in the future, lasers will probably be superior.

See also: Electrolysis, lasers, waxing

Exercise

We exercise to stay fit, healthy, and trim. When done on a regular basis, exercise can enable us to live longer. But does exercise help us look younger? The answer seems to be yes and no.

Say you live in a tropical or desert area and are able to exercise outdoors every day. While exercising will benefit your health, daily sun exposure will age your skin. Without wearing sunscreen or exercising early or late in the day, you can actually look older even though you are physically in shape.

On the other hand, regular toning of muscles helps us fight the gravitational effects of time because firm muscles can limit sagging to a certain degree. Because it promotes circulation, exercise also helps fight unwanted fatty deposits such as cellulite. Regular exercise indoors or when the sun's rays aren't strong seems to be the best way to stay in shape and look younger.

See also: Diet, sun protection, wrinkles

Exfoliators

Our skin is always renewing and replenishing its top layer of cells. Exfoliators help speed up this process by removing dead skin cells and allowing the new skin layer to emerge. Exfoliators do not remove wrinkles or lessen sun-damaged skin. Because they help bring newer skin to the surface more rapidly, the skin will look better. Exfoliators are most often used on the face.

Exfoliators are available over the counter or as procedures in spas and salons. Some over-the-counter exfoliators include moisturizers containing the fruit acid glycolic acid (an alphahydroxy acid), lactic acid (an alphahydroxy acid), and salicylic acid (a betahydroxy-like acid). These products are available in pharmacies, department stores, and salons. Semiabrasive scrubs such as the Buf-Puf, or even mild sanding products, can be purchased over the counter at salons, department stores, and pharmacies. These abrasive scrubs should be used gently so they don't overirritate and burn the skin. Professional salon procedures such as facials also exfoliate dead skin cells. Prescription-strength alpha- and betahydroxy acid products, the antiwrinkle cream Renova, and chemical peels not only exfoliate, but also lessen sun-damaged skin and provide an overall smoother appearance to the skin.

See also: Alphahydroxy acids, betahydroxy acids, Buf-Puf, chemical peels, facial masks, facials, Renova

Eyebrow lift

If you feel your face is always looking angry or worried, you may want to consider having a plastic surgeon perform a brow lift. Sagging eyebrows are the result of genetics and the environment. With time, the effects of gravity, and sun damage, the muscles and skin in your forehead that support the eyebrows lose their elasticity. In rare cases, the eyebrows can even droop down near the eyelids and impair your vision. Brow lifts are also performed to tighten and lift wrinkled, sagging foreheads.

Brow lifts are surgical procedures that may involve the removal of excess skin and muscle tissues. Alternatively, brow lifts can be performed via tiny incisions made in the scalp area above the forehead (without removing the skin) to tighten only the muscle tissue directly below the hairline. In this sense, brow lifts differ from lasers that promote skin regeneration, but cannot remove excess skin.

Different incisions are made for a brow lift. For example, an incision directly above the eyebrow is often best for men who may have hair loss. An incision in this location hides the scar in the natural creases of the forehead just above the eyebrow. However, forehead wrinkles cannot be smoothed by an incision directly above the eyebrows. If you already have natural creases on your forehead, an incision made right in one of these creases effectively hides the scar. In women, incisions are often made in the hair, not only to lift up the eyebrows, but also to smooth out and tighten the forehead skin. Your hair then hides whatever scar may be left from the procedure. Consult a plastic surgeon for the procedure that is appropriate for you.

Brow lift surgery is done with intravenous sedation or general anesthesia and the procedure usually takes less than three hours. After a brow lift, some pain, swelling, and bruising may be expected for a week or two. Temporary numbness and hair loss may also occur in the area of the incision. In order to minimize side effects, you should follow your surgeon's instructions.

A new high-tech approach to the brow lift called the endoscopic brow lift uses long, ultrathin telescopes. During an endoscopic brow lift, the facial plastic surgeon makes a tiny incision at the hair line, places the endoscope underneath the skin and muscle of the forehead, and works down to the area of the eyebrows. Once there, most doctors use special instruments to elevate the muscles above the eyebrow and stitch them in place. The effect is a higher eyebrow, made with one tiny, hidden incision. Forehead wrinkles can also be lifted with this endoscopic procedure.

See also: Face-lift, intrinsic aging, lasers, photo damage

Eyelid surgery (blepharoplasty) *[blef-ar-o-plas-tee]*
Often, sagging eyelids are a byproduct of aging, heredity, sun exposure, and other environmental factors. Even blinking over a lifetime can stretch the skin and muscles enough to loosen them up. Sometimes upper eyelids can droop so far over the eyes that the person can't see.

Blepharoplasty can solve the problem. Performed by facial plastic surgeons and some specialized dermatologists, blepharoplasty removes excess skin from the upper eyelids, lower eyelids, or both, tightening the skin and thus eliminating the bags. Taking only a few hours, the surgery is performed under intravenous sedation or general anesthesia.

The surgeon makes a precise incision that is camouflaged in the crease of your eyelid, then removes the excess, sagging skin and (if necessary) the fat pads underneath the skin. The remaining skin is then finely stitched together. The scars that result are invisible because they will blend into the creases around your eyes. You can expect bruising around the eyes for a week or two, but makeup can be used as camouflage. Most patients are able to return to work after one week.

A newer approach to lower eyelid lifts is called transconjunctival *[trans-con-junk-tie-val]* blepharoplasty. Fatty deposits are removed through an incision made just inside the lower eyelid, in the pink area of your eye, thus eliminating scars on the outer skin. Your facial plastic or oculoplastic surgeon (a surgeon who specializes in eye procedures) can help you decide the best method.

See also: Baggy eyes, face-lift

F

Face-lift

As we age, the face and the neck are subjected to both intrinsic aging, the natural, nonenvironmental effect of time on the skin, and extrinsic aging, the effects of sun damage and environmental factors, such as smoking.

A face-lift is the surgical way to repair sagging skin by tightening areas of the face and neck, especially the lower parts of the face. A face-lift takes approximately two to four hours, performed by facial plastic surgeons. It usually requires intravenous sedation or general anesthesia. Anyone over the age of thirty-five can consider a face-lift, but should consult a facial plastic surgeon.

A face-lift is different from laser resurfacing and chemical peels, which remove the top layers of skin so that wrinkles (especially those around the eyes) are "ironed out" and younger, healthier skin regenerates. By contrast, a face-lift tightens the skin by pulling it up; the body does not regenerate any new skin.

In order to tighten the skin on your face (and sometimes neck), the surgeon makes incisions through the skin, raises it up, and repositions it so it is tighter and looks firmer. The excess tissue is then removed. Although all surgical procedures leave scars, a skilled plastic surgeon hides scars from a face-lift so they are not really noticeable. In women, scars are usually hidden in the hairline and the creases of the ears. In men, scars can be hidden in the hairline and in the sideburns.

After the procedure, dressings and bandages are placed on the face for several days. Some redness, bruising, and swelling can be expected for a few weeks. Most people take one to two weeks off work to recuperate. It is very important you follow your plastic surgeon's detailed instructions.

As face-lifts do not prevent the sun and time from imposing their effects on your skin, future tuck-ups may be necessary if your skin starts to become loose again. You should minimize sun exposure and also use skin-care products recommended by your dermatologist or plastic surgeon.

See also: Chemical peels, intrinsic aging, lasers, photoaging

Facial hair

The desirability of facial hair depends upon one's age, gender, and culture. A young man with a baby face often feels that a beard will help him look older. By contrast, a more mature man with a receding chin or hair line may feel that a beard will help him look younger. In men, beard growth occurs most rapidly around age thirty. As they age, some women grow facial hair on their chin, upper lip, or in the sideburn area.

Male receding hairlines and female facial hair can be caused by the same process. Both men and women have dihydrotestosterone, a form of the male hormone testosterone, in their blood. If this hormone level is increased the hair follicles will be affected and facial hair in women and baldness in men will result. The increase in hormone levels is usually not even measurable on a blood test. What is puzzling is that this increase in dihydrotestosterone causes hair follicles in one location, the scalp, to fall out, and in another, the beard area and upper lip, to grow.

Methods to remove unwanted facial hair include shaving, waxing, electrolysis, and lasers. Shaving is an easy, quick, and painless way to remove unwanted facial hair; however, the fast regrowth of hair requires the procedure to be repeated frequently.

Women usually have both hot and cold waxing done in a salon or spa. Waxing is especially popular for chin, eyebrow, and sideburn areas, and for upper lip hair removal. Waxing can be painful and carries a risk of burning the skin, sometimes so severe that treatment by a dermatologist is needed. However, a wax buffered by soothing agents is now available in some salons for those who have sensitive skin. Another small risk is follicle infection. Hairs removed by waxing do grow back, but much more slowly than shaved hair.

Electrolysis is a procedure that usually results in permanent hair removal. Electrolysis is painful and time consuming: the electrologist uses a magnifying glass to detect each individual hair before eradicating it. Often, only twenty-five to seventy-five hairs can be treated in one visit, so multiple visits are necessary to complete hair removal in just one area. However, if a person has only a few upper lip, chin, or sideburn hairs to remove, electrolysis represents an attractive choice.

Lasers are much less painful than all of the above procedures—and significantly faster. They work by targeting the pigment cells that are located on each hair beneath the skin, and often it takes only a few treatments to remove the unwanted hair permanently. The success of lasers to permanently remove excessive hair is comparable to that of electrolysis, but in the future lasers will probably be more effective.

See also: Electrolysis, excessive hair, lasers, waxing

Facial masks

Masks have always been used to maintain a more youthful appearance. Masks are based in wax, rubber, oatmeal, and mud. They can be purchased over the counter, or applied in salons, spas, and some dermatologists' offices. In general, masks are left on the face for ten to thirty minutes.

Wax-based masks are made from beeswax or a combination of paraffin and a petroleum jelly-like material. This is usually applied hot. They are most helpful for people with dry skin because the wax acts as a physical barrier so that water does not evaporate from the face.

Rubber-based masks can be purchased over the counter. The mask is usually squeezed out and then applied to the face. This mask makes the skin feel as if it has been tightened. It will also feel soft and refreshed. They are safe for dry, normal, combination, and oily skin types.

Oatmeal-based facial masks are mixed with water to make a paste. They can help normal or combination skin. They leave the skin feeling soft, smooth, and tightened.

Mud masks are made of absorbent clay. They have an astringent-like effect. Oily pores and acne-prone skin benefit the most from these.

Facials

In a typical salon facial the skin is analyzed and cleansed. Blackheads and whiteheads are extracted. The skin is massaged and then at least one mask is applied, then the skin is hydrated with a moisturizer or protective cream.

The most important outcome of a good facial is skin so clean you can't achieve the like at home. Deep-cleansing facials exfoliate the skin in order to bring healthy, fresh skin to the surface. Often a low-strength glycolic acid peel or enzymatic peel with papaya or pineapple is included to aid in the exfoliation process. The most common type of facial currently in vogue is called a European facial, so named because of the particular massage technique used. The massage not only relieves tension, but may improve circulation as well. Some aestheticians believe that relaxation of facial muscles through massage may minimize the appearance of wrinkles.

See also: Facial masks

Fat removal

How and where we accumulate fat is often genetically and environmentally determined, but as we age our bodies tend to accumulate fat. Men and women are encoded differently genetically and metabolically, and so their "fat sites" seem to be predetermined by their sex: men tend to gain weight around their stomachs, and women tend to gain weight around their hips, thighs, and buttocks. While diet and exercise play a role in firming and toning the body, removing unwanted fatty deposits is often accomplished by a variety of procedures and products, including liposuction, Endermologie, and thigh creams, all with varying results.

Liposuction is performed by a specialized dermatologist or plastic surgeon who inserts a small metal tube attached to a pumplike device into the unwanted fat sites to literally suck out the fat. Common areas of treatment for men include the "love handles" on the waist; for women it is the thighs, calves, hips, waist, or area under the chin. Liposuction is not a substitute for proper diet and regular exercise, but is helpful for people who have specific areas of fatty deposits they want eliminated. For more information on this technique, see Liposuction on page 88.

Endermologie is a process that purportedly thins thighs by rolling them in a massaging device that smoothes the cellulite and thus promotes good circulation. Sessions with the Endermologie technique, when coupled with regular exercise and a low-fat diet, may help firm the fat on thighs. Endermologie is performed by some dermatologists and plastic surgeons. Some spas offer the service, and some physicians use Endermologie in addition to liposuction. Many spas combine a variation of the Endermologie technique (utilizing massage), as well as heat packs and herbal pastes to eliminate the appearance of cellulite. The herbal wraps may consist of natural ingredients, such as lemon, green tea, fennel, algae, kola nut, and ivy. These procedures have not been proven effective, although some aestheticians and dermatologists advocate their results.

Over-the-counter thigh creams are products advertised to help firm fat. Usually these are based on herbs, botanicals, or the caffeine-like ingredient in coffee, methylxanthine *[meth-il-zanth-eene]*. There is no scientific evidence demonstrating these creams have any more than a minimal effect on fat reduction.

See also: Cellulite, liposuction, thigh creams

Fat transplantation

If you have prominent creases between your mouth and cheek, or between the chin and cheeks, you may want to fill them in by having fat transplantation. This procedure is different from using a synthetic filling substance such as Gore-Tex, or a human tissue bank material like Alloderm, because unlike other fillers, fat transplantation uses your own fat taken from an inconspicuous place to fill a wrinkle. In a way, fat transplantation is similar to Autologen, as both procedures transplant material for the benefit of filling wrinkles. Autologen, however, uses your body's collagen, while fat transplantation involves the use of your biological material below the collagen layer in the skin, called the fat layer. Because fatty tissue is bulkier than collagen, fat transplantation is used to fill very deep folds in the skin, while Autologen is best reserved for smaller wrinkles. This procedure is performed by specialized dermatologists and plastic surgeons.

A local anesthetic is administered before some of the fat (usually from the hip area) is removed through a syringe. The doctor then removes any blood residue from the fat and prepares the fat to be injected into the area of the face. After injection, your depressed area often appears overly swollen, and temporary bruising may also occur. There is no risk of an allergic reaction to your own fat, so no allergy testing is necessary, as with Collagen injections. The injected fat is eventually absorbed by the body, so you will need touch-up injections.

See also: Alloderm, Autologen, chin implants, Collagen, deep wrinkles, Gore-Tex

Fibrel

Fibrel used to be commonly used by dermatologists and plastic surgeons to treat depressed scars and fill wrinkles.

However, because of recent production problems as well as the abundance of other readily available wrinkle-filling materials, it is not commonly used today.

Fibrel is a liquid substance made mainly from gelatin. The gelatin compound fills the scar or wrinkles and is reported to stimulate collagen growth. Fibrel is injected through a syringe into or under the small depressed areas of the skin. Its effects generally last about a year. Because there is a slight risk of an allergic response, an initial skin pretest with Fibrel is important.

Fibrel does not work on all scars and is no longer often recommended to fill deep or fine wrinkles.

See also: Autologen, Collagen

Fine wrinkles

Fine wrinkles are lines that occur on the skin as we age. Also called small wrinkles, they result from a natural loss of the skin proteins collagen and elastin. However, fine wrinkles can also come from exposure to the sun. In short, both intrinsic aging (due to time and genetics) and photoaging (due to sun exposure) are characterized by fine wrinkles.

They can be treated by smoothing or filling them out. Glycolic acids, the antiwrinkle cream Renova, and chemical peels are used to smooth out and reduce fine wrinkles. Erbium:Yag and CO_2 lasers are used to smooth out fine wrinkles more thoroughly. Collagen and collagen-like products are used to help fill out fine wrinkles.

See also: Intrinsic aging, photoaging, small wrinkles

Fluid intake

There is an old adage that drinking eight glasses of water a day helps keep the skin moisturized and young looking. The truth is that while drinking a lot of water is good for the body in general, water intake does not directly affect how fast the skin ages. On the other hand, proper and daily use of moisturizers on the skin make the skin look softer, hence younger looking. Your dermatologist can explain how to use moisturizers.

See also: Moisturizers, wrinkles

Free radicals

First proposed in the 1950s, the free radical theory of aging assumes that free radical production is directly responsible for age-related changes that occur throughout the body. Today, many scientists believe in this theory, as there is an increasing number of research studies that demonstrate the damage which these dangerous compounds are responsible for.

Free radicals are toxic molecules formed from air pollution, smoking, and sun exposure. Because they are inherent in our environment, it is hard to avoid coming into contact with them. They are unstable, especially reactive atoms or compounds that have one or more unpaired electrons. (Normally, oxygen is a stable molecule with paired electrons, but a free radical oxygen atom has unpaired electrons.) It can wreak havoc on the skin by destroying the normal function and integrity of other neighboring molecules. It can even damage the DNA that carries our genetic code. Such changes in our molecular structure age us and can eventually cause cancer. Once balanced, they no longer threaten our health.

When rubbed on your skin or taken as a pill, antioxidants reduce or eliminate the harmful effects of free radicals. (Antioxidants rubbed on the skin are primarily effective on free radicals produced by the sun.) In essence, they provide a stable atomic home for these unstable molecules. Common antioxidants are vitamin C, vitamin E, the enzyme catalase, the enzyme superoxide dismutase, and beta-carotene, a form of vitamin A. Doctors agree the best way to enhance your antioxidant health is to eat plenty of fresh fruits and vegetables and take vitamin supplements.

Although research about antioxidants is in its infancy, their action as barriers to the potentially cancerous results of free radicals seem to justify their widespread current use.

See also: Antioxidants, intrinsic aging, photoaging

G

Glycolic *[glie-kol-ik]* **acid**

Glycolic acids are the most widely used form of alphahydroxy acids. Low-strength formulations for acne treatment, pore refinement, and exfoliation are available over the counter at spas, salons, and pharmacies. They usually contain less than 10 percent "free" acid—that is, the amount of acid that works on your skin. Glycolic acid may be the only active ingredient in a preparation or may be combined with a moisturizer.

Prescription-strength agents generally contain 10 to 20 percent free acid and may be obtained from a dermatologist. Some studies indicate that products with a stronger glycolic acid content increase the flow of blood to the skin and thereby promote the growth of new skin cells and collagen, a natural skin protein. This in turn helps improve sun-damaged skin more than the exfoliation produced by the lower-strength, over-the-counter products.

In addition, after several months of application, the stronger-prescription glycolic acids reduce wrinkling and brown, blotchy spots to a minor degree. These acids can be used with the antiwrinkle cream Renova to achieve an even greater reduction of sun damage, including fine wrinkling, provided they are applied at different times of the day.

How do glycolic acids compare to Renova? Consistent application of glycolic acids will improve your skin; however, some dermatologists believe topical prescription-strength glycolic acid is roughly only half as effective as daily Renova use.

Glycolic acid is also available in "lunchtime peels." Salon-strength, glycolic acid peels are not as effective or strong as those applied at a dermatologist's office. While peels are much stronger than topical preparations, they need to be repeated every few weeks. Some dermatologists feel it's best to use a daily regimen of skin rejuvenation products such as glycolic acids and/or Renova before starting glycolic acid peels. The combination can enhance the effect of each peel.

See also: Betahydroxy acids

Gore-Tex

Over the past thirty years, Gore-Tex has been used by vascular surgeons to patch blood vessels. Today, dermatologists and plastic surgeons make use of this synthetic material to patch and fill the deep wrinkles and crevices in the face. Gore-Tex is primarily used to fill in prominent lines at the junction between the mouth and the cheek, thick frown lines, and lines in the cheeks, or to thicken lips. It is available in millimeter-thin strips, or as a threadlike material.

After local anesthesia, a doctor makes two tiny incisions on either end of the wrinkle. With a special threading device onto which the Gore-Tex is attached, the doctor inserts the material into one end of the incision and pulls it out through the other. The threading instrument is then detached from the Gore-Tex, leaving the Gore-Tex in the skin, filling the wrinkle.

Although a very safe synthetic material, temporary side effects include bruising and swelling, along with a very slight risk of infection and scarring. The Gore-Tex implant lasts approximately five to fifteen years, and occasionally requires adjustment after implantation. This implant is also removable.

See also: Alloderm, cheek implants, fat transplantation, lip enhancement

H

Hair loss

Among adults, the most common kind of hair loss is called androgenetic alopecia *[an-dro-gen-e-tik al-o-peash-a]*, otherwise known as male- and female-pattern hair loss. It is characterized by large, normal-length hairs becoming smaller, very fine, and almost microscopic. After a number of years, these tiny hairs may fall out, even to the point of permanent loss. Androgenetic alopecia is a genetic problem, and the testosterone family of hormones, present in both men and women, is thought to play a major role in its cause. Androgenetic alopecia is initiated by an abundance of the testosterone derivative dihydrotestosterone *[die-hie-dro-testos-ter-own]*. Although they are chemical cousins, testosterone and dihydrotestosterone have different functions in the body, and only dihydrotestosterone promotes androgenetic alopecia.

Men are visibly more affected than women by androgenetic alopecia because their hair loss is more noticeable on the *top* of their heads and the sides of the frontal region, known as "widow's peaks." In women, a "widened part" occurs centrally on the scalp, but the hairline on the front does not recede and the hair at the forehead line remains intact.

Many treatments are available today to help lessen androgenetic alopecia. These include nonprescription topical solutions, prescription pills, cosmetic procedures such as hair weaves, and surgical treatments, such as hair transplants.

The most commonly used over-the-counter topical medication is minoxidil, available in 2 and 5 percent solutions. Although it is not proven, minoxidil is thought to stimulate hair growth by altering chemical transport around the hair cells, thereby causing hair cells to proliferate. Studies show that minoxidil can generate some hair growth (which seems to reach its maximum potential after six months of use); however, it seems to be more effective on women than on men. Overall, the percentage of people who respond to minoxidil is limited.

The most common prescription men use to restore hair is Propecia pills. The introduction of Propecia represents a significant advance in the treatment of androgenetic hair loss in men. And, for the first time, scientists have marketed a pill that attacks hair loss at its known chemical origin. Propecia prevents dihydrotestosterone from signaling the hair follicles to shrivel up. Propecia seems to work only on the hormonal influences at the top of the scalp; other hairs on the sides of the scalp, face, and body are unaffected by it. In clinical trials, a definite increase in hair growth starts after six months and continues to grow for at least two more years.

Propecia is for men of all ages and for women who no longer want to have children. Because it blocks the male hormone dihydrotestosterone, it is possible that boys born to women who are taking Propecia would be feminized. There are other medicines like Propecia that are currently being tested by scientists and will probably be available shortly.

Spironolactone is a pill often used by women with androgenetic alopecia. Spironolactone is a diuretic that in lower doses has the effect of blocking dihydrotestosterone. Hair regrowth with spironolactone is a slow process, as it takes at least six to twelve months to take effect. Spironolactone cannot be given to men because it may stimulate breast enlargement. Spironolactone is not approved by the Food and Drug Administration as a treatment for female hair loss, and thus its use by dermatologists is called "off label." Discuss this medicine carefully with a dermatologist before starting therapy.

At salons and specialized centers, hair weaves and additions are often performed to cover up hair loss. Both real and synthetic hair can be attached firmly to the scalp. Some methods of attachment include weaving the new hair with existing hair, applying adhesives, suturing, and the use of hair clips. Most of these attachments can be well hidden.

Hair transplantation is performed by specialized dermatologists and plastic surgeons. Hairs from the sides of the scalp are grafted in small amounts at a time and placed where you want hair to grow. Hair transplantation is a slow process, and usually requires multiple visits to your physician.

Transplanted hair may not look natural for several months while it grows out, and surgical touch-ups are often necessary. In general, men over fifty with lighter-colored hair and skin and a more advanced state of baldness gain the most from hair transplantation. Although rare, risks include scarring, formation of tiny skin cysts, and gel-like blood deposits under the scalp. A temporary numb feeling and infection may also occur in the areas treated.

See also: Hair transplantation

Hair transplantation

Hair transplantation is the process of surgically relocating hair. Hairs from the sides of the scalp are grafted in small amounts to places where you want hair to grow. Miraculously, these hairs are not aware of the relocation, so they respond to hormones in the same way as if they were still on the side of the scalp. Because of this, transplanted hairs do not usually miniaturize or fall out.

Hair transplantation is a slow process, usually requiring multiple visits to your physician. Local anesthesia and localized blocks at nerve roots are used to prevent pain. Some scabbing and redness on the scalp are to be expected after surgery. While it grows out, transplanted hair may not look natural for several months. Surgical touch-ups are often necessary since most people continue to lose other scalp hair as they grow older.

In general, older men benefit more than younger men from hair transplantation because their hair loss has stabilized—they will not lose much more hair in the future. For similar reasons, balder men benefit because they have less additional hair to lose after the transplant is completed. Scalps that have lighter hair and skin color provide a better color match and also blend better with the transplanted hair. Some procedural risks include scarring, formation of small skin cysts, or gel-like blood deposits under the scalp. A temporary numb feeling and infection may also occur in the areas treated. Hair transplants are performed by specialized dermatologists and surgeons.

See also: Hair loss

Hormone creams

Normal hormonal balance is an essential part of health and well-being, although hormone levels can change as we age. One study found that women going through menopause have less collagen in their skin. Conversely, the women who took hormonal replacement therapy lost less collagen.

(Collagen is a skin protein that helps maintain the skin's strength; if lost, wrinkles can result.)

Researchers are questioning whether a hormone cream rubbed into the skin can maintain healthy collagen, or perhaps even promote its growth. Unfortunately, the answer is still unclear. There have been a few scientific studies that demonstrate a slight improvement in skin thickness and collagen content from estrogen (female hormone) cream rubbed into the skin, but these studies have not been replicated. Hormone creams are usually purchased over the counter. A dermatologist can determine the usefulness of a hormone cream for your skin.

See also: Ethocyn

I

Intrinsic aging

Intrinsic aging refers to changes that occur in the skin solely due to the passage of time. By contrast, photoaging refers to the cumulative effects of sun exposure on the skin. Intrinsically aged skin can have fine or small wrinkles, a loose or sagging quality, and skin growths that do not become cancerous. For example, take a look at the skin on your buttocks or inner surface of your arm, both of which have not had much sun exposure. Unlike photoaged skin there are no deep wrinkles, or irregular color and texture.

Most of today's antiaging products focus on sun-damaged skin; however, many can be used to lessen the effects of intrinsic aging as well. Renova is a Food and Drug Administration-approved cream that diminishes the appearance of fine wrinkles, minimizes brown irregular blotchiness, and smoothes out the skin's texture. Prescription-strength alphahydroxy acids also improve texture, tone, and wrinkles on the skin. Chemical peels, laser resurfacing, face-lifts, and wrinkle-filling substances are more complicated methods used to lessen the effects of aging.

See also: Alphahydroxy acids, chemical peels, face-lift, lasers, photoaging, Renova

Isolagen *[ice-all-a-jen]*

Isolagen is a liquid substance that is injected by a tiny syringe into deep wrinkles or depressed scars, similar to the way Collagen, a cow-derived form of human collagen, and Dermalogen, a reconstituted form of human collagen, are injected. Frown lines and lines around the mouth are favorite sites for the use of Isolagen. Because Isolagen is made from your own skin, there is virtually no risk of an allergic response.

To create Isolagen, a dermatologist takes a tiny piece of skin from around your ear, leaving a very small scar. The skin is sent to the Isolagen laboratory to be separated by cell type. That is, the cells that manufacture collagen in your body are separated from other skin cells and stimulated to grow in the lab. The full-grown cells are then sent to the dermatologist as a liquid that can be injected into your skin. In essence, you now have your own collagen-making cells filling your wrinkles.

Because the new collagen-producing cells take time to naturally create a collagen matrix, the effects of Isolagen are not visible for months. In fact, you never know if the injected cells will grow to make collagen at all. By contrast, Collagen, Dermalogen, and Autologen are prepared collagen-like materials, and thus blend with your skin immediately. However, if Isolagen works, your deep wrinkle may stay filled in much longer than with other products. This lasting effect has not been proven scientifically as yet.

See also: Autologen, Collagen, deep wrinkles, Dermalogen

J

Jessner's peel

A Jessner's peel uses a combination of chemicals to achieve a skin peeling between superficial and medium depth. Over forty years ago, Max Jessner, M.D., wanted to combine several low-strength peeling agents into one chemical peel. He combined salicylic acid and lactic acid with other chemicals. Today, some dermatologists still use it to treat acne or diminish wrinkles. However, the glycolic acid peel has reduced the use of Jessner's peel. Jessner's peel is not available commercially and must be prepared by a pharmacist if a dermatologist decides to use it. A dermatologist can help you decide if a peel with Jessner's formula is appropriate for you.

See also: Chemical peels

K

Kinetin *[kine-a-tin]*

One way to smooth and soften the skin, and reduce the brown irregular spots and small wrinkles on your face, may be a product with Kinetin. Kinetin, an ingredient in some over-the-counter creams and lotions, slows aging in plants and enhances plant growth. Researchers in the Kinetin laboratory initiated a study to see if the compound would have the same effect on people. At the end of six months of daily Kinetin and sunscreen use, scientists noticed a slight reduction of irregular brown spots and a softening to the skin's texture.

Kinetin products can be compared in strength to over-the-counter products such as retinols and alphahydroxy acids, which make the skin feel softer and smoother. The effectiveness of a Kinetin regimen compared to prescription-strength alphahydroxy acids and Renova cream is unknown.
See also: Alphahydroxy acids, fine wrinkles, photo damage, Renova, sun damage

Kogic acid *[ko-jik acid]*

Kogic acid is a gel applied directly to the skin over several weeks. It diminishes or eliminates unwanted pigmentation. Kogic acid can also be used on sun freckles, small areas of skin discoloration, such as melasma, or on the pigmentation remaining after acne has healed.

Kogic acid is effective because it acts on the pigmentation compound that makes up brown spots. However, it can be irritating to the skin, and must be carefully applied. If not, the spot can actually look worse than it did before treatment. In fact, usually kogic acid is not combined with other brown-spot-reducing creams like Retin-A because of an increased potential for irritation.

Kogic acid is available from some dermatologists and plastic surgeons in prescription-strength form, but is not available in pharmacies. It is sometimes sold in a much weaker form at spas and can be a minor ingredient in cosmetics sold over the counter.

See also: Bleaching creams, melasma, Retin-A

L

Lactic acid

Like glycolic acid, lactic acid (which comes from sour milk) is a naturally occurring alphahydroxy acid. In fact, Egyptians are said to have bathed in sour milk to make their skin softer. Lactic acid creams have been used for years to smooth and moisturize the skin, and to lessen the rough, irritated skin (which is inherited) that occurs on some persons' arms and legs. Both glycolic acid and lactic acid creams have also found new applications.

Some dermatologists feel that lactic acid may work as well as glycolic acid in improving sun-aged skin. There is some scientific evidence to support this claim, but most dermatologists feel that the evidence remains inconclusive. Lactic acid creams (in strengths of ten percent or less) are available over the counter at your pharmacy and a twelve percent cream is available by prescription.

A new thirty percent lactic acid cream, called Lac-Hydrin 30, is currently awaiting FDA approval and should be available by prescription (from your dermatologist) very soon. Because of the higher concentration of lactic acid, Lac-Hydrin 30 appears to be more effective than lactic acid in lower concentration and also may be more effective than any glycolic acid creams currently available. During much of the 1990s, the makers of Lac-Hydrin 30 have conducted rigorous, large-scale scientific studies in order to prove to the FDA that their product lessens some of the features of photoaging, such as fine wrinkles.

When approved, Lac-Hydrin 30 will join Renova as the only creams to satisfy the FDA that they reverse some of the sun aging process. More information about Lac-Hydrin 30 will become available during the next few years as both scientists and the public gain experience with this latest addition to fight aging skin.

See also: Alphahydroxy acids, betahydroxy acids, glycolic acid, photoaging, wrinkles

Large pores

Large pores seem to be inherited. They can increase as we age, and they tend to cluster around the nose and central part of the face. In general, pores are openings for oil glands and hair follicles. There is currently no permanent way to eliminate them, but there are many ways to help reduce them.

Over-the-counter toners and astringents can help dry the skin, and remove excess oils from pores. Glycolic and salicylic acids, in over-the-counter creams and in more potent chemical peels, help reduce large pores. Prescription creams like Renova and Retin-A are also helpful.

See also: Renova, salicylic acid

Laser dermabrasion (laser resurfacing)

Laser dermabrasion, better known as laser resurfacing, has completely changed the character of dermabrasion: most dermatologists have switched from using traditional dermabrading instruments to lasers.

Laser resurfacing was made possible when scientists modified one of the earliest lasers, the CO_2 laser, to emit shorter, more controlled superpulses for precision performance. The high-frequency superpulsed CO_2 lasers vaporize microscopic layers of skin cells so that the depth of penetration can be closely controlled. Even with this greater control, however, the superpulsed CO_2 laser still penetrates the skin deep enough to make it comparable to a deep chemical peel or to the traditional method of dermabrasion, which carry some risk.

Like dermabrasion and deep chemical peels, CO_2 laser resurfacing is recommended only for people with at least a moderate amount of wrinkles and sun-damaged skin. With the CO_2 laser, you can resurface the entire face or just the areas around the eyes or mouth. This laser can also be used to smooth out deep acne scars. Intravenous sedation is necessary, and you can expect the healing process to take up to several months. In general, resurfacing with the CO_2 laser is preferable to older dermabrasion methods.

After CO_2 laser resurfacing, the face is very raw looking and may be scabbed, primarily due to the fact that sun-damaged skin has been removed and the new skin needs time to grow and regenerate. Strict adherence to the laser surgeon's guidelines is necessary during the recovery period.

Over the past few years, the Erbium:Yag laser (Erb:Yag for short) was developed for more superficial resurfacing than the superpulsed CO_2 laser. The Erb:Yag laser does not penetrate as deep as the CO_2 laser, so that patients can have fewer layers of skin removed. The recovery period with the Erb:Yag laser is shorter, usually under two weeks, and some redness and scabbing occurs. Often, only topically applied or injected anesthesia is needed with the Erb:Yag laser. It is recommended for people who want more wrinkle reduction than a chemical peel offers, but less wrinkle reduction than a CO_2 laser offers.

Several months following CO_2 laser resurfacing, some people may have a recurrence of blotchy brown pigmentation, or they may experience persistent redness. In rare instances scarring occurs. Many scientists believe that lighter-skinned people tolerate laser resurfacing and heal better than darker-skinned people. Laser dermabrasion is not always permanent, and sun-damaged skin can recur after several years.

See also: chemical peels, CO_2 laser, deep wrinkles, dermabrasion, Erbium:Yag laser, lasers, photo damage

Lasers

Due to technological advances, the use of professional lasers for skin-care improvement has mushroomed from its beginning twenty years ago, and many laser systems are now available.

Laser stands for "light amplification by stimulated emission of radiation." A laser beam is a uniform, unidirectional beam of only one wavelength of light energy, created when gases (such as carbon dioxide) or crystals (such as ruby) are stimulated with electricity. The light emitted through these gases and crystals carries a specific, single wavelength of light energy that can target its object. Typically, lasers in use today get their name from the element that is used, such as Ruby, Alexandrite, Erbium:Yag, and Neodymium:Yag.

Medical lasers work in a unique way: coherent light waves specifically target certain components of the skin and leave surrounding skin components unharmed. In this context, the "surrounding skin" includes the layers above and below the area of skin the dermatologist wants precisely improved or eliminated. Today, the laser system a dermatologist selects is driven by the need for a particular wavelength of light, which will effectively destroy only the target area on or underneath the skin.

Laser researchers soon realized that a specific wavelength of light energy could be absorbed uniquely by one component of the skin but not another. This means that the laser may not touch the surface of the skin, but will reach below it. The pulse dye, or vascular, laser reflects this principle. It emits a single wavelength of light visible as yellow light that is toxic to components of the blood; if you were to point a laser beam made of one wavelength of yellow light at a container holding some blood, only the blood will be destroyed, not the container. Because yellow light does not destroy parts of the skin that do not have blood, it will travel harmlessly through the skin cells and tissue above and around the blood. Dermatologists can treat any blood-filled spot with this laser, such as broken blood vessels, spider leg veins, spider veins on the face, cherry angiomas, hemangiomas, and other unwanted red-colored spots on the skin.

Similarly, there are now lasers that can target the pigment cells in the skin in an attempt to remove unwanted pigmented spots without harming the surrounding skin. This technique is a little more challenging, however, because all skin has some degree of pigmentation. Thus, occasionally the laser can remove too many pigmented cells in a brown spot, and leave it as a white spot. This is especially true for darker-skinned people.

The Neodymium:Yag, Alexandrite, and Ruby lasers are used to remove unwanted pigmented spots (pigmentation after a rash has healed, sun freckles, melasma), unwanted tattoos, and unwanted hair. These lasers remove excessive hair by targeting the pigment cells that are near that part of the hair where growth occurs.

By contrast, the wrinkle-removing lasers, namely the superpulsed CO_2 and Erbium:Yag lasers, emit a single wavelength of light that destroys anything with water in it. The superpulsed CO_2 laser is an advanced form of the older, original CO_2 laser. The Erbium:Yag laser is a variation of the Neodymium:Yag laser but does not target pigment cells because the addition of the element erbium changes the laser's wavelength to target water. As the skin has water in it, these lasers vaporize and remove targeted wrinkled skin on contact. These two lasers are different from the original CO_2 laser, which also targeted water, because they emit very precise, short pulses that allow skin removal to occur rapidly, but still virtually eliminate collateral damage to surrounding skin. The Erbium:Yag laser does not penetrate or remove skin as deeply as the superpulsed CO_2 laser, and hence it is used to remove more superficial wrinkles.

Risks are specific to the type of laser used, but may include prolonged redness and scarring as with the CO_2 laser, or blotchy brown pigmentation as with the Alexandrite and pulse dye lasers.

What lies in the future for laser technology? In the upcoming decade, dermatologists will have a "tunable" laser, where all of the lasers we use will be combined into one unit. On entering a specific colored wavelength, a physician will be able to eliminate the target area of skin that needs to be altered, whether it is a blood-colored growth, or the top layers of facial skin.

See also: Alexandrite laser, CO_2 laser, deep wrinkles, Erbium:Yag laser, Neodymium:Yag laser, Ruby laser, spider veins, sun freckles

Lip enhancement

If you think your lips are thinner than they used to be, you may want to contact a dermatologist or facial plastic surgeon to make your lips fuller.

One of the older methods we still use is Collagen, derived from cows. No anesthetic is necessary. Today, collagen-like substances such as Dermalogen can also be injected to fill out lips. These methods are not permanent, and touch-ups are required.

Implants, such as Alloderm and Gore-Tex, can permanently fill the lips in one treatment. Alloderm, a collagen-like substance made from human skin, and Gore-Tex, a synthetic material, both come in very thin sheets that a doctor shapes and inserts into the lips with a special instrument. Procedures with Gore-Tex and other similar synthetic materials are reversible, so if you do not like the result or position of the implant, it can be removed or repositioned.

A surgical procedure called lip advancement can also make your lips fuller. Performed with local anesthesia or mild sedation, the red inner part of the lips (on the inside of the mouth that lies against the teeth) can be moved, "advanced" farther on the skin that surrounds the lip. The skin that has been advanced over is removed, so the result is an enhanced lip. The incision made in this procedure is hidden at the border of the new, and fuller lip. Recovery from lip advancements usually takes less than a few weeks.

See also: Alloderm, Collagen, Dermalogen, Gore-Tex, SoftForm

Lipoic acid *[lie-po-ik asid]*
Lipoic acid is an antioxidant compound that soon may be found in products sold in pharmacies and natural health stores. (Antioxidants help our bodies destroy harmful free radicals produced by environmental toxins.) Lipoic acid can be used as a cream or a pill. Scientists in Germany recently noted that lipoic acid not only works as an antioxidant, but also prevents another antioxidant, vitamin E, from being depleted after skin is exposed to harmful ultraviolet sun rays. In essence, it is an antioxidant that protects other antioxidants.

It is also possible that lipoic acid reduces wrinkles. However, to date, this effect is based on observations of only one dermatologist. Nevertheless, as an antioxidant, lipoic acid, like vitamins C and E, appears to have strong sunscreen-like ability. In the near future, many sunscreens or other products that offer sun protection may contain lipoic acid to enhance their effectiveness.

See also: Antioxidants, free radicals, vitamin C, vitamin E

Liposomes
Liposomes can theoretically make a single product penetrate the skin nine to fourteen times more effectively than it would on its own. Liposomes can be compared to a laser guidance system on a smart bomb that enables the bomb (or medication) to reach its target area more efficiently. The liposome delivery system prevents the medication from being absorbed elsewhere in the body, so that the topically

applied cream or medication works without interruption on the target areas.

Liposomes were first discovered by chemists in the 1960s. Chemists have had difficulty in keeping them stable enough to work. Understandably, both cosmetic and pharmaceutical industry scientists have been busy doing research on liposome delivery systems in topically applied preparations, such as creams, moisturizers, cosmetics, and some antiaging medications. Hopefully, liposomes in the future will significantly extend the effectiveness of these products.

Liposuction

One of the more common surgical procedures performed today, liposuction eliminates cellulite and other fatty areas of the body. Developed in France and brought to the United States approximately twenty years ago, liposuction provides a quick fix for those people with have areas of fatty deposits they want eliminated in one outpatient procedure. In men, this often includes the love handles around the waist, or a double chin. In women, bulging thighs, hips, waist areas, and neck are most often treated.

Specialized dermatologists and plastic surgeons perform liposuction. A skilled physician inserts a small metal tube into the site of the fat. When this instrument is attached to a pumplike device and placed within the fatty areas of the body, it literally sucks out the fat.

Originally, patients were administered general anesthesia for liposuction. This made it costly, and carried risks arising from general anesthesia. Liposuction performed with the patient asleep also created a large amount of blood loss. Sometimes even blood transfusions became necessary.

Today, liposuction is primarily done with the tumescent *[too-mess-ent]* technique developed about fifteen years ago by a Southern California dermatologist, Jeffrey Klein, M.D. Tumescent means "firm and swollen." Dr. Klein discovered that a numbing medicine diluted in a large volume of saline solution (the salt solution that makes up our body fluids) made liposuction possible without general anesthesia and the large blood loss associated with it. The saline-diluted numbing medicine is inserted in the fatty areas targeted for removal. The area swells and becomes numbed—the patient has no sensation there. The physician then removes the fat with this small metal tube attached to a pump. During a tumescent liposuction you can actually can talk with the doctor, read a book, or watch television while your fat is being removed. Blood loss is minimal because the large amount of saline placed in your body reduces the risk of bleeding. The numbing medicine also helps prevent bacterial infection.

After tumescent liposuction, the areas where the fat was removed remain swollen, due to the saline fluid inserted before the procedure. Over the next several weeks it is necessary to wear a special pressure garment that helps absorb the fluid as it leaks out through the skin. Also, temporary bruising occurs at the site of the injection. It is critical that the patient follow the doctor's aftercare instructions.

More uncommon risks include gelled blood deposits (hematomas) under the skin, thick fluid deposits under the skin (seromas), and infection. On occasion, the liposculpted areas may stay numb for several weeks or months. Before making arrangements for this surgery, consult a dermatologist or plastic surgeon who has sufficient experience with this process.

See also: Cellulite, fat removal

M

Mask of pregnancy

The common name for the medical term melasma, or mask of pregnancy, refers to brown spots that appear under and around the eyes and on the cheeks while a woman is pregnant. It appears that the combination of hormonal changes during pregnancy and sun exposure produce these irregular brown spots. It does not require much sun exposure for this mask to appear.

See also: Melasma

Masks (see facial masks)

Melanin

Melanin is the pigment that is responsible for the color of skin. Small amounts of melanin are found in light-skinned people, such as Caucasians; moderate amounts are found in somewhat darker-skinned people, such as Hispanics and Asians; and greater amounts are found in darker-skinned people, such as African Americans. The darker the skin color the more protection the skin has from the sun. There is a lower incidence of skin cancer, sun-damaged skin, and wrinkles in darker-skinned than in lighter skinned people.

Some research indicates that melanin works as an antioxidant to destroy the harmful free radicals that arise when sun rays strike the skin. Melanin can now be synthesized in the lab. It can be added as an ingredient to sunscreen and moisturizer preparations to further protect the skin from the sun. Melanin applied directly to skin does not tan or even darken it. Melanin is just beginning to be used in over-the-counter products. In the future many more products will probably contain melanin.

See also: Antioxidants, photo damage, sunscreen

Melasma *[mel-az-ma]* (mask of pregnancy)

Melasma (the mask of pregnancy) is triggered by exposure to the sun. It often occurs in pregnant women or in women who take birth control pills. Once on your face, melasma may stay after childbirth or birth control pills are discontinued. Common sites for melasma include the upper lip (many people feel they have a "chocolate mustache"), under the eyes, and on the upper cheeks.

Interestingly, melasma looks a lot like some brown spots or freckles from sun exposure. In general, dermatologists use the same methods to treat melasma as they treat other sun-related brown discolorations and blotchiness. The most common treatment is a prescription bleaching cream used with or without the antiwrinkle cream Renova and the antiacne cream Azelex. If the areas of melasma are small, they can be treated with the pigment gel kogic acid (purchased at a dermatologist's office) or with a direct freezing spray. Lasers that specialize in removing brown pigment are also used to remove melasma, including the Ruby, Alexandrite, and Neodymium:Yag laser. If your melasma covers a fairly large area, chemical peels can be used to help lighten the darker pigmentation. These peels are often used in combination with nightly creams like Renova or alphahydroxy acids and bleaching creams. Wearing sunscreen on a regular basis helps prevent melasma from becoming worse. Consult your dermatologist to determine the advantages and disadvantages of each of the above treatments.

See also: Azelex, bleaching creams, chemical peels, kogic acid, lasers, photoaging, Renova, salicylic acid, sun freckles

Melatonin

Melatonin is a hormone made in the pineal *[pie-neel]* gland of the brain. In both animals and humans, the levels of this hormone decrease with age. In some studies, when melatonin supplements were given to animals, they had a longer lifespan. Consequently, some people believe that by taking this hormone as a daily supplement they will live longer. Melatonin is available over-the-counter. Some people use it in place of a prescription sedative. Before you try melatonin, it is probably best to discuss it with a doctor, as its health risks are unknown.

Moisturizers

Overly dry skin may not only be unattractive, but also uncomfortable. Dry skin looks and feels rougher and older than oily or normal skin. Dry skin is especially noticeable in the winter because the air is colder and less humid (unless you live in a state like Florida). Moreover, when you're inside the house in wintertime and the heat is on, your skin becomes drier.

The face has a large number of oil glands that keep our faces moisturized, but oil gland production often decreases as we get older, and occasionally even the face can become as dry as the skin on the rest of the body.

The solution is constant use of moisturizers sold at salons, spas, department stores, and pharmacies. The type you choose depends on how dry your skin really is. For example, you probably want to use a lighter moisturizer on your face than on the rest of your body. Many people use a light moisturizing lotion on their bodies during the summer and a heavier one during winter.

Lighter moisturizers are called lotions; they contain a high content of water (look at the first ingredient on the label), so they evaporate quickly and soon leave the skin feeling dry. Heavier moisturizers contain more petrolatum and less water. In fact, one of the heaviest moisturizers is pure petroleum jelly. Because it does not evaporate quickly it protects the skin from drying out for a very long time.

Most people do not need something as thick as petroleum jelly, so moisturizing preparations often combine petrolatum and water in close to equal amounts. These moisturizing compounds are called creams.

Moisturizing creams can also contain an additional ingredient, referred to as a humectant *[hue-mek-tant]*. Humectants help bring moisture from below the skin up to the skin's surface where it is needed. One common humectant is glycerin. A good moisturizing cream contains a humectant to bring moisture up to the skin and a petrolatum mix just thick enough to trap that moisture. A dermatologist can help determine which moisturizer best fits your skin type.

See also: Dry skin

N

Neodymium:Yag laser

Yag is an acronym for yttrium-aluminum-garnet laser, the elements that give this laser its unique qualities. There are two types of Yag lasers: the Neodymium:Yag (called Nd:Yag) and the Erbium:Yag (called Erb:Yag). When dermatologists speak of the "Yag laser," they are alluding to the Neodymium:Yag laser.

The Nd:Yag laser emits a wavelength that targets brown- and black-colored areas on and under the skin. The Nd:Yag was originally developed to help remove tattoos, but technological improvements allow it to be used for the removal of unwanted brown spots, such as the sun freckles on faces and on the backs of hands and forearms. The Nd:Yag laser is used to remove unwanted hair. Side effects include temporary scabbing and bruising. Uncommonly, a lightened spot can occur if too much pigment is removed.

By contrast, the Erbium:Yag laser smoothes out fine lines and wrinkles. The wavelength is changed so that this emitted light is absorbed by any skin, whether it has a pigment or not. Because all skin is affected, it is considered a resurfacing laser. Some swelling, redness, and scabbing may occur after the treatment—it is better to take a week or two absence from work.

See also: Alexandrite laser, Erbium:Yag laser, hair removal, lasers, Ruby laser

Nutrition

Good nutrition is important for good skin tone and texture. As we grow older, changes in the gastro-intestinal tract can lessen absorption of nutrients, even if we eat a balanced diet. Overall signs of malnutrition can include dry skin, itching, brittle nails, and hair loss. Older individuals can be deficient in zinc, copper, iron, vitamin B6, thiamin, vitamin K, vitamin A, and folic acid. Lack of vitamin A can cause dry, plugged hair pores on the arms; lack of vitamin K can cause bruising. Since we do not know if deficiencies (no matter how small) in these nutrients accelerate the aging process, it may be wise to take a daily vitamin supplement after a certain age.

Some alternative medical practitioners offer nutrient injections and infusions, as they believe these added nutrients help us keep our vitality and youth. Any vitamin supplementation should be discussed with your doctor.

See also: Diet

P

Phenol peel

Phenol peels penetrate more deeply into the skin than superficial glycolic acid peels and medium-strength trichloroacetic acid (TCA) peels. Phenol is an acid which is used diluted as a disinfectant (carbolic acid). Phenol chemical peels are comparable in strength to laser skin resurfacing using the CO_2 laser, and are best reserved for people who want to remove a lot of sun-damaged skin and deep wrinkles and who are able to take several weeks off from work while they recover. Like the superpulsed CO_2 laser, phenol peels are useful in helping reduce acne scarring as well as unwanted brown spots. Unlike lasers, phenol peels have been performed by dermatologists and plastic surgeons for over thirty years. The effect of a phenol peel is long-lasting, and does not require repeated treatments.

The pain from a phenol peel is similar to the pain from CO_2 laser resurfacing. Therefore, intravenous sedatives or anesthesia is necessary. After applying the phenol peel, petrolatum is usually applied to the skin for forty-eight hours. There are two potential risks in getting a phenol peel. Your heart has to be monitored during the procedure because heart damage may result. There is also a possibility of kidney damage. Intravenous fluids are usually used. Phenol peels are usually done in several sessions, and take anywhere from sixty to ninety minutes. One can expect severe redness, peeling, and sometimes scabbing after a phenol peel, as it takes at least several weeks to regenerate younger healthy-looking skin. You must follow very specific aftercare instructions from your physician to reduce side effects. Uncommon side effects include increased blotchiness, long-lasting redness, and scarring.

See also: Chemical peels, laser dermabrasion, photo damage

Photo damage

Photodamaged skin is the medical term for sun-damaged skin, also known as photoaged skin. Photoaging differs from intrinsic aging that is unrelated to the sun and environment. Compare the skin on your face with your buttocks (a place that is not usually exposed to the sun) to see the difference between intrinsic and photoaged skin. The total process of aging is called extrinsic aging—which adds to the cumulative effects of intrinsic aging, photoaging, and environmental aging (the result of environmental exposure, such as cigarette smoke or smog).

Photodamaged skin is rough, loose, wrinkled with small and deep crevices, and has irregular brown pigmented spots. Precancerous and cancerous growths occur on photodamaged skin. Small broken blood vessels called telengectasia *[tel-an-jek-taze-ya]* may also be present. In people of Celtic origin, photoaged skin may appear more ruddy and thin, and have many telengectasias.

One of the reasons photo damage is so prevalent these days is because the American culture incorrectly associates tanned skin with a healthy, youthful glow. Over a century ago, tanned skin was associated with the working poor who were exposed to the sun as they labored outdoors. The wealthy stayed indoors, as fair skin was considered healthy and pure. However, times have changed. Now most people work inside, so a sign of wealth is to head south, bask in the sun, or enjoy a day at the beach or poolside. In fact, it is said that up to 50 percent of photo damage today occurs before we turn twenty.

Fortunately, a revolution about how to reverse and prevent photoaging is occurring. People are starting to realize the value of protecting themselves and their children from the sun by daily use of sunscreen. In the laboratory, antioxidants are being combined with sunscreen to further enhance effectiveness. Antiaging creams are available over the counter and by prescription. Lasers and surgical procedures can also help reduce the damage caused by the sun. Tanning creams that stain the skin with a tanned look are available and are safe and look natural. In the future, a tanning cream may be available that will cause the skin to actually tan without being exposed to the sun's rays. For more information on how to improve photodamaged skin, please see the entries listed below.

See also: Alphahydroxy acids, face-lift, intrinsic aging, lasers, Renova, sun protection

Photoaging (see photo damage)

Placenta extract
A placenta is the fetus's carrying sac while still developing inside its mother's uterus. Components of human and animal placentas are often referred to on cosmetic containers as "placenta" or "placenta extract." It is said that placenta extract enhances blood flow to the skin and helps cells grow and function. In order to prepare placentas for cosmetic use, they are churned up, frozen, and rinsed with sterilized water. Additional modifications and processing may be required depending on its ultimate cosmetic use, which vary

from hair conditioners to facial moisturizers. The benefits of placenta extract have yet to be scientifically proven.

Power peel

In a power peel, a machine that uses a tiny stream of aluminum oxide crystals gently removes the top layer of dead skin cells from someone's face. This procedure, termed a microdermabrasion by dermatologists, is relatively painless, and not really "powerful" at all. Multiple power peels may reduce some signs of sun damage, such as fine wrinkles, and are an alternative to alphahydroxy and betahydroxy acid peels. They are performed at the dermatologist's or plastic surgeon's office, and at some salons.

See also: Chemical peels

Pulse dye laser (vascular laser)

The pulse dye laser was the original laser developed during the 1980s to treat red skin discoloration. Also called the vascular laser because it selectively targets blood vessels, the pulse dye laser can be used to treat red and purple birthmarks on the body and telengectasia (small blood vessels) that can develop on the face from sun damage, rosacea (an inherited skin condition), or trauma. A special form of the pulse dye laser is used to treat spider veins on the legs. The treatment is much less painful now that newer lasers have a cooling device to decrease the sensation of the laser on the skin. A visible purple bruise usually develops and can last from seven to ten days, although the cooling device helps limit this side effect.

See also: Lasers, spider veins

R

Red spots

A common complaint among people visiting their dermatologists is the desire to "get the red out" of their skin. Small red bumps and dots, also known as cherry angiomas, often develop on our skin as we age. Small, red threadlike blood vessels called telengectasias *[tell-ang-jec-taze-yas]* can also develop on the face, neck, and chest over time, especially if we have had a fair amount of sun exposure.

Factors unrelated to aging or sun exposure, such as pregnancy and hormones, seem to contribute to the production of cherry angiomas. They can be removed with an electric needle called a cautery, or lasered off with the pulse dye laser. Sometimes when they are large, a dermatologist will choose to remove them with a scalpel and then stitch the skin. Telengectasias on the face, chest, and neck can also be removed with the electric cautery needle or pulse dye laser. *See also:* Cautery, pulse dye laser, spider veins

Renova

If you want to ameliorate the aging effects of the sun, Renova cream is the treatment of choice. Renova helps smooth and soften the skin, while lessening fine lines and decreasing any brown blotchiness on your face. Prescribed by your dermatologist, Renova is the only Food and Drug Administration (FDA)-approved medication that can decrease the ravaging effects of years of sun exposure. None of the other prescription or prescription-strength creams discussed in this book carry the FDA seal of approval for this purpose. (Lac-Hydrin 30 is currently awaiting FDA approval as a cream to lessen sun-damaged skin. See the entry "Lactic acid" for further details.)

What is Renova and why is it the only antiwrinkle cream to gain FDA approval? In the 1980s, dermatologists and their patients realized that the vitamin A-derived Retin-A cream could treat more than just acne. Many people began to notice that when they used Retin-A for acne their faces became smoother, softer, and less wrinkled. The word rapidly spread. Unfortunately, Retin-A can be very drying and irritating to adults with dry skin.

The manufacturers of Retin-A realized that if they could change the base ingredients of Retin-A to make it more moisturizing, while retaining the active ingredient (called tretinoin *[tret-in-o-in]*), they would have a great "antiwrinkle" cream. They also realized that in order to gain FDA approval, large scientific studies would be required to prove its effectiveness in improving wrinkles and other aspects of photodamaged skin. A new moisturizing cream of Retin-A was devised, and was named Renova.

Renova was studied for several years and given to thousands of people by selected scientists across the country. It was learned that Renova reduces fine wrinkles, diminishes brown spots and irregular brown blotchiness, and smoothes and softens the skin by an average of 20 to 30 percent after six months of nightly use. Renova doesn't do this merely by exfoliating the skin—it actually causes new, healthy collagen to form as well. In other words, it can make the skin look younger by rejuvenating its "roots." Further studies have also shown that after one year of nightly Renova use, you can use it just two to three times per week for maintaining your improved look. Because Renova underwent all of this rigorous scientific testing, the FDA gave its approval in 1996 for it to be marketed as a prescription cream designed to lessen the effects of sun-damaged skin.

For the first few weeks of its use, Renova causes some dryness and peeling, especially around the mouth. Your face then adjusts to the cream's active ingredients. If peeling persists beyond several weeks or if your skin is sensitive, Renova may not be your best choice.

Renova is applied at night after removing any dirt and makeup before retiring. Because there is a special way to apply it, you will need to discuss its application and benefits with your dermatologist. Using Renova requires the use of a daily sunscreen, or a moisturizer and sunscreen combination.

Renova can also facilitate procedures such as laser resurfacing and many types of chemical peels. The preparation for these procedures involves using Renova nightly for several weeks beforehand. Renova can also be used with a glycolic acid (at different times of the day) to enhance its effect. *See also:* Alphahydroxy acids, chemical peels, fine wrinkles, lasers, photo damage, Retin-A, sun damage

Restylane

Restylane gel is a filling agent used to treat prominent wrinkles and crevices. Used in Europe for over five years, Restylane should soon be available in the United States. Restylane is produced from a material called hyaluronic *[hie-a-loor-on-ik]* acid, a natural component of the skin that helps it remain firm and thick. Like the trademarked Collagen, Restylane is injected directly into the wrinkles.

Like Collagen, it can be used for fine and deep wrinkles. Occasional touch-ups will be needed. Because it is synthetically made rather than animal derived, as with Collagen, there is no risk of an allergic reaction.
See also: Collagen, Dermalogen, fine wrinkles, Isolagen

Retin-A

A prescription cream that has been used by teenagers with acne for the past thirty years, Retin-A gained its fame during the 1980s when dermatologists became aware that this medicine smoothes out wrinkles. The manufacturers of Retin-A then sponsored scientific studies to prove that the active ingredient in Retin-A indeed did reduce wrinkles and other effects of sun damage. Retin-A was then reborn as Renova, a cousin with the *same* active ingredient (tretinoin *[tret-in-o-in]*), but with a moisturizing base. The base makes Renova more suitable for adults and less useful for oily-skinned and acne-prone teenagers. Today, Renova is used instead of Retin-A for decreasing wrinkles and other features of sun-aged skin.
See also: Renova

Retinol

Retinols are vitamin A-derived cream-based products that are used to repair the signs of sun-damaged skin. Retinol creams were originally developed in the 1950s to treat acne and acne-related disorders, but scientists found Retinol creams to be unreliable because they were inactivated quickly when applied to the skin. Scientists substituted the active Retinol molecule for a similar, but more stable compound, tretinoin *[tret-in-o-in]*, and created Retin-A, a very effective antiacne cream that has been used for years.

Due to increases in technology, scientists have discovered a way to keep Retinol creams chemically active and useful. In the last five years, Retinol creams have been sold without a prescription and marketed to help reduce the signs of aging. Retinol creams are available at pharmacies, salons, and department stores. Some dermatologists' offices offer it in a cream base which utilizes microsponge technology, a "time-release" method.

Although Retinol creams may help reduce some aspects of sun damage on your face, it is still unclear how well these creams really work. Retinol creams have not been compared to glycolic acid creams or Renova to determine whether it is as effective as these more established products.

See also: Glycolic acid, photoaging, Renova, Retin-A

Ruby laser

A versatile laser with multiple uses, the Ruby laser is named after the ruby crystal that helps give it the unique wavelength of visible light it emits. The Ruby laser is used to lessen unwanted brown spots such as sun freckles and melasma, and remove tattoos and unwanted hair. Moreover, the Ruby laser is often "quality switched," to give it increased strength.

Because treatment methods with the ruby laser are somewhat painful, dermatologists often use local anesthesia prior to treatment. Slight redness and scabbing usually occur after each treatment. The Ruby laser carries a slight risk of leaving a light-colored or darker-colored mark on the skin after the healing is complete.

See also: Lasers

S

Sagging earlobes

Loose, sagging earlobes probably result from a combination of factors, including heredity, sun exposure, and heavy earrings. Earlobes have less firm tissue than other parts of the body, so they tend to sag more easily. Sagging earlobes are an indication that the normal fat cells in the earlobes have been replaced by a fatty residue that is less firm.

To correct these, a relatively short procedure, called a z-plasty, can be performed by a facial plastic surgeon. The treatment leaves a small scar that usually blends into the surrounding skin. This procedure requires only local anesthesia.

Sagging skin

Why does the skin seem to loosen and sag with age? First, the older we become, the more time for the force of gravity to work. Gravity works much like a small dead weight. Muscle tone diminishes over time, as our previously firm faces and bodies will sag as the flesh hangs from the muscle. Sun exposure adds to the problem, making the skin looser and more wrinkled. Years of cumulative sun exposure carves a leathered, but loosened, look on our faces. This phenomenon is quantified by the decreased amount of collagen in sun-damaged skin.

Luckily, there are many procedures today that can help us defy Father Time. Face-lifts can pull the face tighter; eyebrow lifts can help sagging foreheads and eyebrows; and liposuction can help tighten up our abdomens and other sagging, fatty areas of the body. Collagen and other synthetic materials like Gore-Tex can be injected or implanted into sagging cheeks to firm them up. Thus, sagging skin can be surgically tightened and removed, or filled up, to look more youthful.

See also: Aging, cheek implants, eyebrow lift, eyelid surgery, Gore-Tex, liposuction

Salicylic *[sal-a-sil-ik]* acid

Physicians have used salicylic acid for decades to treat childhood and teenage acne, primarily blackheads and the large pores that often accompany acne. Chemically, salicylic acid is classified as an "aromatic" acid, and is somewhat similar to betahydroxy acids.

Over-the-counter salicylic acids are still sold under the name "betahydroxy acids," even though that label isn't entirely accurate. These cream or lotion products can help exfoliate the skin and improve blackheads and large pores. They are available at salons, department stores, and pharmacies. It is not known how salicylic acid products measure up against glycolic and other alphahydroxy acids that are available over-the-counter.

During the 1990s, the uses of salicylic acid expanded, as it arrived on the antiaging market in creams and chemical peels to help reduce wrinkles and enhance a youthful appearance. They are named "lunchtime peels" because you can have the peel done during your lunch hour, return to work, and have few, if any, noticeable side effects. These superficial chemical peels make your face smoother and softer, diminish irregular brown pigmentation, and reduce fine wrinkles. Marketed as the BETA-Lift x peels, superficial

chemical peels with salicylic acid seem to work about as well on sun-damaged skin as superficial chemical peels that contain glycolic acid, but many dermatologists feel that the BETA-Lift x peel is easier to use and produces a more predictable effect than glycolic acid peels. Superficial salicylic acid peels are also excellent acne reducers as well.
See also: Alphahydroxy acids, betahydroxy acids, chemical peels, melasma, photoaging

Sclerotherapy *[sklair-o-ther-a-pee]*
Sclerotherapy removes unsightly leg veins that tend to surface as we age. A dermatologist or vascular surgeon injects a liquid compound directly into the veins you want eliminated, causing blood vessels to shut down. Sclerotherapy can be done on small, thin "spider" veins as well as on varicose veins. Sclerotherapy on larger, more prominent varicose veins is often performed with ultrasound guidance techniques, whereby an ultrasound probe is used to locate the varicose veins for easy injection.

Saline and sodium tetradecyl sulfate are the two most commonly used sclerosing compounds in the United States. Saline, a natural fluid component of the body, is generally safer, as there are fewer possible side effects and the risk of an allergic response is nonexistent. Saline used in sclerotherapy is much more concentrated than the saline fluid in the body; when injected into a blood vessel, it causes the blood vessel's walls to be destroyed. Saline works well on smaller spider veins, but has little effect on larger vessels.

Sodium tetradecyl sulfate is usually more effective than saline, and works on spider veins as well as larger vessels.

Because it is detergent-based, it destroys blood vessel walls more rapidly than saline. However, with sodium tetradecyl sulfate there is a greater possibility of side effects and a very small risk of an allergic response. Uncommon side effects include redness, bruising, light brown spots that look like freckles, small ulcers, and the appearance of very tiny blood vessels around the sites where the veins were. Consult your dermatologist for the method best for you.

See also: Pulse dye laser, spider veins

Small wrinkles

Small wrinkles occur as part of the normal aging process, called intrinsic aging. Therefore, small wrinkles occur on skin areas that are exposed to the sun and those areas that are not. Small wrinkles are usually most prominent around the eyes, but they can be present anywhere.

After several months of nightly use, prescription-strength creams like Renova and glycolic acids reduce and smooth out small wrinkles. Superficial chemical peels and Erbium:Yag laser resurfacing are the most common procedures used to smooth out small wrinkles. Although primarily used for deeper wrinkles, medium-strength deep chemical peels and CO_2 laser resurfacing also remove small wrinkles. Collagen injections and other similar filling substances can fill in small wrinkles, making them as smooth as the rest of your skin. Consult your dermatologist for which treatment is best for you.

See also: Chemical peels, Collagen, fine wrinkles, intrinsic aging, lasers, photo damage, Renova, wrinkles

Smoking

Fortunately, smoking is not as popular as it used to be, as it contributes to the aging process in the face. The effects of smoking are often visible as deep wrinkles around the mouth area. Even exposure to second-hand smoke causes wrinkles. Cigarette and tobacco smoke are known to cause cancer both internally and on the skin. When it comes into contact with the body tissues, tobacco smoke triggers free radicals (toxic molecules), which can permanently damage our cells. Mutations and other cellular abnormalities result, contributing to increased risk of cancer and the formation of wrinkles. These changes begin to appear after many years of smoking.

See also: Free radicals, wrinkles

Smoothing

Rough skin often occurs as part of the aging process when skin has had periods of extensive sun exposure over many years. Smoothing our skin, especially our faces, makes us look and feel younger. When the skin is smoothed, the dead skin cell layer is exfoliated, leaving only the newer cells on the surface.

Exfoliating the skin, with nightly use of over-the-counter glycolic and salicylic acids, is an effective way to achieve softer and smoother skin. Many different brands are available, and it's best to select one that your skin feels most comfortable with. Your dermatologist can also recommend specific brand names. Facials and some facial masks performed by a licensed aesthetician also leave the skin feeling smoother and softer. In addition, prescription-strength glycolic acid creams and prescription creams like Renova smooth and exfoliate the skin. Chemical peels and laser resurfacing are more involved procedures that also exfoliate and smooth your skin.

See also: Buf-Puf, chemical peels, facial masks, facials, glycolic acid, lactic acid, lasers, Renova, salicylic acid

SoftForm

A synthetic implant that has been used for a quarter of a century in general surgery to repair damaged blood vessels and hernias, SoftForm is a thin, tubular-shaped material made to fill the deep creases that have formed on your face. After local anesthesia, a dermatologist or plastic surgeon places SoftForm through a thin incision at one end of a deep wrinkled crevice. The SoftForm implant is then pushed through the crevice underneath the skin, exiting through another thin incision made at the other end of the deep crevice. SoftForm is most often used for deep frown lines or creases around the mouth, or into the lips (for fuller lips). Some temporary redness and swelling are possible side effects. Initially, one can feel the SoftForm implant underneath the skin, but after several months it is usually less noticeable to the touch. SoftForm implants are permanent, but the procedure is reversible and there is no risk of an allergic reaction.

See also: Alloderm, deep wrinkles, Gore-Tex

SPF (sun protection factor)

SPF stands for sun protection factor, and the acronym is used to convey how much protection a sunscreen gives.

Actually, SPF measures only the amount of sun protection from the burning ultraviolet B rays, and does *not* measure protection from ultraviolet A rays. (Both ultraviolet B and A rays contribute to aging of the skin and skin cancer.) The higher the SPF number on the bottle of sunscreen, the more protection there is from the sun's ultraviolet B rays. As a rule of thumb, any sunscreen with an SPF of less than 15 will not provide much sun protection. For extended sun exposure for more than two hours, an SPF of at least 30 is recommended by most dermatologists. Because SPF measures only protection against ultraviolet B rays, it is advisable to make sure that the label of the sunscreen you buy also indicates it has ultraviolet A protection.

There is currently no ratings system for ultraviolet A rays protection, but one is in the final stages of development.

See also: Photo damage, sun damage, sun protection, sunscreen

Spider veins

Spider veins are the thin little veins that sometimes radiate from a central area, like a spider's legs. While the exact cause of spider veins is unknown, several factors seem to contribute to their appearance. The fact that spider veins occur more in woman than in men suggests that female hormones may be a contributing factor. Moreover, women who take birth control pills and other female hormone supplements seem to have an even higher incidence of spider veins. It is also known that spider veins tend to increase during pregnancy. Certain families are predisposed to getting spider veins, suggesting a hereditary influence.

Trauma to an area on the leg can lead to spider veins occurring in that area at a later time. Standing on your feet for a long period of time and heavy weight-bearing exercise also induce spider veins.

Scientists have not yet found a way to prevent the formation of spider veins, but wearing compression hose, if you are on your feet a lot, and regular aerobic exercise, seem to help. Dermatologists eliminate spider veins with a procedure called sclerotherapy *[sklair-o-ther-a-pee]*, which involves injecting a solution into the spider veins. These solutions, containing either concentrated saline or sodium tetradecyl sulfate, work by shutting down the blood flow to the spider veins. Common side effects after sclerotherapy include bruising and small freckle-like brown spots at the sites of injection. The bruises disappear after several days, but sometimes the spots can last a long time. Rare side effects, more common with sodium tetradecyl sulfate, include small ulcers, redness, and infection. After sclerotherapy, you may need to wear support or compression hose for a specified time.

During the past five years, some pulse dye lasers have been especially designed to eliminate spider veins. These lasers have hand pieces specifically designed to fit over spider veins. They also have "cooling tips" that make the procedure virtually painless and may reduce the common side effect of bruising. Some dermatologists feel that the improved pulse dye laser is as effective as standard sclerotherapy for eradicating spider veins on the legs.
See also: Red spots

Sun damage

Sun damage contributes significantly to the formation of wrinkles. Cumulative sun exposure over prolonged periods of time contribute to what dermatologists call photoaging. Damaged by the sun's ultraviolet rays, photoaged skin can have a rough texture, irregularity of color and tone, wrinkles, fine, threadlike blood vessels (called telengectasias), and brown spots called sun freckles.

Wearing a daily sunscreen or moisturizer containing a sunscreen is the best way to prevent sun damage. Luckily, we have ways today to reverse or remove some of the effects of sun damage. Renova is the only Food and Drug Administration-approved prescription antiwrinkle cream that has been shown to reverse sun damage to some extent. When used nightly for several months, prescription-strength glycolic acid creams can also reverse some of the sun damage. Chemical peels and laser resurfacing performed by the dermatologist or facial plastic surgeon can also help. Your dermatologist can help you decide which treatment is best for you.

See also: Alphahydroxy acids, bleaching creams, chemical peels, kogic acid, lasers, photoaging, Renova, salicylic acid, sun protection, sunscreen

Sun freckles

Also called "liver spots," sun freckles are the brown, irregular stains that occur on the parts of the body exposed to the sun, such as the face, arms, and hands. They are not usually considered dangerous, but on very rare occasions can become cancerous. There are several approaches to removing sun freckles, including freezing with a very cold spray, using kogic acid, lasers, or bleaching creams. The antiwrinkle cream Renova may also help reduce sun freckles. None of these methods guarantee complete removal of the freckles, and each method occasionally leaves the spot either darker or too white. Your dermatologist can help you determine which treatment method is best for you. *See also:* Bleaching creams, kogic acid, Renova

Sun protection

Dermatologists always recommend sun protection for all of their patients, regardless of age. Why is this? The sun's ultraviolet rays cause toxic molecules called free radicals to form in our skin, wreaking havoc by destroying the normal function and integrity of neighboring molecules. As such, they damage our cells' DNA, and damaged DNA can lead to cancer. Whether your skin has been sunburned or sun-tanned, it has been damaged, and repeated episodes of excessive sun exposure will irreversibly damage your skin. The signs of sun damage, such as wrinkles, sun freckles, and brown pigmentation will appear, and skin cancer may occur. It is therefore important to protect yourself and your children from the sun at an early age.

The simplest form of sun protection is wearing the proper clothing. Hats that really block the sun can protect much of your face. Thicker white and light-colored cotton clothing provides better protection than thinner, darker clothing. Some companies, such as Sun Precautions, offer catalogs filled with tested, sun-protective clothing.

Second to protective clothing, sunscreen is the most important way to shield yourself from the sun. Women can use a moisturizer with sunscreen or sunscreen alone before applying their makeup every day. (Makeup with sunscreen does not usually spread evenly enough to be considered an effective method of sun protection.) Men can use a moisturizer with sunscreen or sunscreen after shaving. When spending more than a few or more hours in the sun, sunscreen should be at a sun protection factor (SPF) level of 30, contain an ultraviolet A ray (UVA) blocking agent, and be applied at least thirty minutes before going out into the sun. Repeat applications every few hours are necessary. (SPF refers to ultraviolet B ray [UVB] protection only, so a sunscreen purchased needs to state that it offers UVA protection as well.)

Antioxidants such as vitamin C and vitamin E also seem to offer sun protection, primarily because they destroy sun-induced free radicals. For example, daily use of a vitamin C cream may aid in sun protection. A sunscreen combined with an antioxidant cream would offer even greater sun protection.

Scientists are now studying topically applied chemical compounds, namely CM-Glucan and 2-FDO (2-furilodoxime), as agents to protect the skin from the sun. Experiments suggest that when 2-FDO is combined with an SPF 4 sunscreen, it becomes equivalent to an SPF 30 sunscreen. Many doctors believe that 2-FDO reduces sun damage by neutralizing the iron that acts as a catalyst to the production of free radicals. In the future, 2-FDO may be widely used to enhance the effectiveness of sunscreen. At present, neither 2-FDO or CM-Glucan are available for commercial use.

An exciting development on the horizon is a tanning cream that actually tricks the skin into tanning, rather than staining the skin (as do currently available tanning creams), by making the skin respond as if it were actually exposed to sunlight. The result is a natural tan without any cost to the skin's vitality. You will be able to work in the morning, apply your cream at night, and come to work the next day with a real tan. And best of all, you do not have to expose your skin to the sun's harmful rays in order to achieve it.

See also: Antioxidants, photo damage, sunscreen

Sunscreen

Sunscreen is one of the most important ways to maintain a youthful appearance. The earlier in life you start using a daily sunscreen, or moisturizer that has a sunscreen in it, the less wrinkled and healthier your skin will look when you are older. Like your daily vitamins, sunscreen is preventative medicine to keep you healthy because it prevents the sun's harmful rays from damaging your skin.

The chemicals in sunscreen agents either interact with skin to prevent the sun from burning it, or physically block the sun, much the way a glove protects your hand from the sun. Blocking agents are less common than chemical sunscreens. Chemical sunscreens contain ingredients that are quickly absorbed by the skin, so you don't even know they are working. They can also be waterproof as well as sweatproof. There are two different types: those with ultraviolet B ray protection only, and those that additionally provide protection against ultraviolet A rays. (Ultraviolet B rays are the burning rays of the sun, but both Ultraviolet B and A rays contribute to skin cancer, wrinkles, and other indicators of sun damage.) The higher the SPF number is on the sunscreen label, the more protection you have against the burning ultraviolet B rays of the sun. In general, the best protection is found in a waterproof chemical sunscreen that is labeled with an SPF greater than 30 and also indicates that it offers protection against ultraviolet A rays.

Physical-blocking sunscreens, like body armor, protect the skin by blocking the sun's rays from ever reaching the skin's surface. Originally, sun-blocking agents, made from zinc oxide, were white pastes that were visible on your skin. Remember a lifeguard with a white paste on his nose? During the last ten years, advances in microtechnology have allowed these zinc oxide preparations and their counterparts, titanium dioxide creams, to be rubbed into the skin. These high-tech physical blocking sunscreens can also be quite water resistant, but not as waterproof and sweatproof as chemical sunscreens can be. Because of their function as an armor, physical sunscreens block all of the sun's rays, whether they are ultraviolet A or B. Physical blocking sunscreens are most effective when the ingredient silicone is added to them.

Any sunscreen should be applied for at least thirty minutes before you go out in the sun, and reapplied every few hours while you are outside. Use sunscreen liberally on your skin, or it won't provide sufficient protection. For example, you need between one-half and one teaspoon to cover your face, one teaspoon on each limb, and up to two teaspoons each on the front and back of your trunk.

See also: Photoaging, sun protection, titanium dioxide, vitamin C, zinc oxide

T

TCA (trichloracetic *[try-klor-asee-tik]* **acid)**
Used in peels by dermatologists for many years, trichloracetic acid (TCA) is a liquid chemical that helps reduce the effects of sun-damaged skin, such as wrinkles and irregular pigmentation. TCA is also commonly used by dermatologists to remove precancerous growths caused by sun exposure. TCA is considered a medium-depth chemical peel, but varies depending on the concentration your dermatologist uses.

The dermatologist applies TCA to the skin with a large cotton swab, or brush. After several minutes a white "frost" appears where the TCA is applied. Because these peels are uncomfortable, most dermatologists recommend an oral sedative prior to the procedure. During the next few days, the skin peels and may look scabbed and red. As with other chemical peels, specific aftercare instructions must be followed.

In general, it takes from several days to two weeks for skin to recover from a TCA peel. The lower-concentration TCA peels have a quicker recovery time, but do not usually remove as much sun-damaged skin as the higher concentrations. Your dermatologist can help you determine which strength TCA is best for you.

When healed your skin will have a newer, healthier look, showing less sun damage. Infection or scarring rarely occurs. The outcome of treatments using liquid TCA is not consistent. To make TCA more reliable, the Blue Peel was developed; it's a paste, not a liquid.
See also: Blue peel, chemical peels

Teeth

No one needs to emphasize the importance placed today on having a beautiful smile. Aside from aesthetic considerations, stained, chipped, and noticeably worn teeth make people appear older than the are; conversely, healthy teeth create the impression of youth.

With age, teeth darken more readily from exposure to coffee, tea, tobacco, juices, and cola. Stains can also be caused by old, defective dental fillings, tooth nerve damage, or trauma to the teeth. Clenching your jaw and grinding your teeth also make your teeth look older. In most people, chipped and worn teeth occur with advancing age. The older the tooth, the more vulnerable it is to chipping and staining.

Fortunately, there is a variety of treatments. A cosmetic dentist (also called a restorative dentist or prosthodontist) can bleach, bond, laminate, and contour teeth to make them look better. The least-invasive treatments include bleaching, bonding, laminating, and contouring.

Bleaching stained or discolored teeth can be performed in the dentist's office or at home, but it is recommended that home bleaching should be performed at the direction of a cosmetic dentist. This treatment, which is most effective on orange, yellow, and brown stains, involves the use of a diluted mix of carbamide peroxide, which is applied in a small, thin, custom mouth guard that is worn for a prescribed number of hours a day (usually during sleep) for two to six weeks. If you persevere, you will enjoy noticeably whiter teeth. Slight touch-ups are usually necessary after a few years. Some people are sensitive to white bleaching, in which case the dentist will change the regimen—usually prescribing the mouth guard for shorter daily sessions for a more consecutive period of days.

Unlike bleach treatments, bonding whitens teeth by the application of small pieces of tooth-colored plastic on the surface of teeth to mask stubborn stains. Bonding is also used to repair chips. Bonding is fairly pain-free, and in most cases patients do not even require local anesthesia. Also, sensitivity is rarely a problem after treatment.

Laminates (sometimes called "veneers") are thin shells made of tooth-colored plastic or porcelain, manufactured in pharmaceutical laboratories. A dentist cements these onto your existing teeth. Laminates can improve the shape and color of teeth, and are particularly effective on moderately worn teeth. The procedure sometimes requires local anesthesia. There should be no post-treatment sensitivity.

Contouring of the teeth involves a slight reshaping by a dentist. This can be done to eliminate small chips, improve old bonding, and enhance the overall appearance of slightly crowded teeth. Usually, no local anesthesia is necessary. If contouring is done sparingly, no postprocedural sensitivity to the teeth should result.

As a general rule, it is a good idea to avoid chewing hard objects such as ice and toothpicks. Not only do these activities cause chipping, they can also ruin the work of even the best restorative dentist. Finally, as with any treatment, it is important to ask your restorative dentist or prosthodontist about the limitations of treatment.

Telomerase

Telomeres are the protective pieces of genetic material at the end of our chromosomes that guard the chromosome from being destroyed. The chemical that keeps these telomere guards healthy is called telomerase. If you lose your telomerase, the guardian telomeres stop working. As we age, our cells lose their telomerase, and one by one we lose our chromosomes, and hence our cells. Some scientists think that taking telomerase pills may save our cells and prolong our lives. Unfortunately, telomerase also promotes cancer. That is, cancer cells are prevented from dying when there is a constant supply of telomerase. Because chromosome-filled cancer cells don't die, taking telomerase may promote cancer.

In the future, the hope for telomerase is for scientists to determine how to preserve telomerase's desirable properties without promoting its negative consequences.

Thigh creams

Thigh creams are over-the-counter creams that contain one or a number of ingredients that help destroy fat deposits, thereby preventing cellulite, or the "cottage cheese" look women often get on their thighs. Caffeine-like compounds are the most common ingredients found in thigh creams, mainly because it is well documented that the caffeine family of chemicals contributes to the slow reduction of fat deposits in the test tube. In people, however, scientific studies have not shown any more than minimal improvement on cellulite with caffeine creams. There are probably two reasons for the discrepancy. First, the reduction of fat deposits addresses only one aspect of the production of cellulite while other contributing factors, such as reduced circulation in the thigh areas, female hormones, and protein deposits, remain unaltered.

Second, the high concentration of caffeine in the cream really needed to break down fat is probably too toxic for human use.

Botanical ingredients, such as sweet clover, ivy barley, lemon, kola nut, fennel, algae, and strawberry, are also believed to help break up cellulite. Botanical cream manufacturers claim their products help disperse toxins and produce a significant reduction in bumpy texture, yet there is no reliable scientific evidence for these claims.

See also: Cellulite

Titanium dioxide

Titanium dioxide is a cream that physically blocks the sun wherever it is applied. Titanium dioxide sunscreens are the most common type of physical-blocking sunscreens currently available. (Sunscreens come in two types: physical-blocking sunscreens and chemical-blocking sunscreens.) Many years ago, titanium dioxide was so difficult to apply that it was not used as much as a chemical sunscreen. Today, due to microtechnology, titanium dioxide is easily rubbed in the skin so that it functions as an invisible shield against the sun. Titanium dioxide is also often found in makeup, but not in a strong enough concentration to have any effect as a sunscreen.

See also: Sun protection, sunscreen

Toners (see astringents)

V

Vitamin A

Vitamin A has been used to treat acne and sun-damaged skin. Vitamin A is also an antioxidant, meaning it lessens or eliminates the harmful effects of free radicals, dangerous molecules that are stimulated and multiplied when the sun's rays strike the skin. A different form of vitamin A, beta-carotene, is found in many green, leafy vegetables, and many believe is as effective as vitamin A.

Accutane is a pill form of vitamin A that is routinely used for extreme acne cases. When used properly, it can be very effective in the control and even prevention of severe cases of acne. Scientific research has also shown that Accutane may help to prevent a few types of cancer. Rare complications include liver damage as well as possible birth defects.

Retin-A and the antiwrinkle cream Renova are topical forms of vitamin A. Retin-A is used to treat acne and Renova is used to reduce the signs of sun-damaged skin. Both medications work by changing the proteins made by your genes so that new, healthier skin is produced. Neither of these topical vitamin A forms should be used if you are pregnant. Consult your dermatologist before using any form of vitamin A.

See also: Antioxidants

Vitamin B

Vitamin B1, B6, B12, and B-complex vitamins have been advertised for stress and are often recommended for women who take birth control pills or suffer from premenstrual syndrome. There have been mixed reports on the ability of vitamin B6 to help the skin. At this point, vitamin supplements of the B-complex variety are not specifically indicated as antiaging remedies.

Vitamin C

Vitamin C has been put into an antiaging cream by several pharmaceutical companies. Dermatologists know that topical vitamin C works effectively as a sun-protecting cream, but, unlike vitamin A products that can reverse sun-damaged skin, the effectiveness of vitamin C to do this is uncertain. Topical vitamin C products combined with sunscreens are currently being investigated by scientists who hope to engineer creams with an enhanced sun-protecting effect. Vitamin C is an antioxidant that inhibits the formation of free radicals, or toxic molecules, thereby protecting the skin against the sun's harmful rays. If vitamin C is taken orally in pill form with vitamin E, it can prevent sunburn.
See also: Antioxidants, Celex-C, sun protection

Vitamin E

Vitamin E is an antioxidant that has been used to help prevent cancer and heart disease by lessening or eliminating the harmful effects of free radicals, dangerous molecules that are stimulated and multiplied when sun rays strike the skin. Recently, vitamin E has been added to moisturizers in an attempt to slow the aging process by preventing free radical formation in the skin. Vitamin E creams have also been touted to expedite the healing of scars, but there is no scientific proof of this claim. A recent study showed that taking vitamin E orally with vitamin C orally helped to prevent sunburn. It is yet to be shown whether this finding correlates with a lower incidence of skin cancer.

Vitamin K

Vitamin K is a mild antioxidant that is now being used topically by dermatologists to reduce the appearance of bruises on the skin. Although current research has not been rigorously controlled, some dermatologists believe that the findings are sufficient to show that topical vitamin K does diminish bruising. Topical vitamin K is especially useful for older individuals who tend to have thin skin that bruises easily. Topical vitamin K is also used to reduce the bruising that occurs after use of the pulse dye laser and for dark circles under eyes. (Topical vitamin K under the eyes often works better when it's combined with a bleaching cream.)

See also: Antioxidants, dark circles under eyes

W

Waxing

Waxing is a procedure usually done in a salon or spa for the temporary removal of excessive hair. Waxing is especially popular for hair removal on the chin, eyebrow, and groin. When the wax is removed from the skin, the hair underneath the wax is pulled out.

Hot waxes are generally made of melted beeswax, whereas cold waxes come in a tube. Sometimes a cloth is placed over the wax so that removing the wax is easier. Some salons use a warm (neither hot nor cold) wax which contains soothing agents for people who have sensitive skin.

Waxing can be painful, and there may be a risk of a burn, sometimes so severe a visit to the dermatologist is required. Another slight risk is the infection of the hair follicles from which hairs have been removed. Hairs removed by the waxing process do grow back, but at a much slower rate than that of shaved hair. Waxing is usually not recommended for users of Renova or Retin-A.

See also: Excessive hair, facial hair

White spots on tanned skin

Have you noticed an irregular brown and white patchiness on your skin? Brown spots intermixed with white spots, particularly on the arms and forearms, are marks of sun damage. The white spots are often more pronounced on tanned skin, because the pigment-making ability of the skin cells there has been impeded.

Protecting the skin by using a sunscreen or covering your arms is essential to prevent the formation of white spots on tanned skin. Prescription-strength glycolic acid creams and prescription antiwrinkle creams like Renova help diminish pigment irregularities caused by sun damage. These creams tend to be more effective on brown spots than white spots.

See also: Photoaging, sun damage

Wrinkles

Wrinkled skin has always been an indication of maturity. Wrinkles are caused by intrinsic and extrinsic factors. Intrinsic aging comes from inherited factors and advancing age processes, while extrinsic aging refers to the cumulative effects of sun exposure, aging, and inherited factors. In general, fine, or small wrinkles are caused by the general aging process and sun exposure. On the other hand, thick, deep wrinkles or furrows are most often caused by repetitive sun exposure which has a cumulative effect on the skin. Deep wrinkles around the lips can also occur from smoking.

As we age, all of us experience some wrinkling, but individuals with more sun exposure over the years will likely develop deeper facial wrinkles as they advance in age. The daily use of a sunscreen or moisturizer along with sunscreen will protect your face from future wrinkles.

Reducing or eliminating wrinkles requires undergoing one of three types of available procedures: You can replace, relax, or remove your wrinkles.

When you have wrinkles replaced, a dermatologist or facial plastic surgeon injects or threads a substance into the crevice of the wrinkle, thereby filling it out, and smoothing it into the rest the skin. Collagen, Dermalogen, and

Artecoll are examples of injectable wrinkle replacers. Gore-Tex, SoftForm, and Alloderm are examples of material inserted to help replace the deeper wrinkles so that the skin can be evened.

Relaxing wrinkles is done with diluted botulism toxin, called Botox. When Botox is injected to relax the muscles that produce the wrinkles, the wrinkles are not so noticeable. Botox can be injected by a dermatologist, a facial plastic surgeon, or an oculoplastic surgeon.

Wrinkles can be removed by a number of methods. Prescription creams like Renova or prescription-strength glycolic acid creams generally reduce fine wrinkles on the face after several months of use. Chemical peels performed by a dermatologist or facial plastic surgeon can also reduce or remove wrinkles. Superficial "lunchtime" peels improve wrinkles, while medium and deep peels can remove wrinkles. Laser resurfacing, also known as laser dermabrasion, is also effective. Your dermatologist can help you decide which method is best for you.

See also: Alphahydroxy acids, Botox, chemical peels, deep wrinkles, fine wrinkles, intrinsic aging, lasers, photoaging, Renova

Z

Zinc oxide

Sunblocks like zinc oxide prevent the sun's rays from penetrating the skin by blocking and reflecting ultraviolet rays rather than absorbing them. Unlike chemical sunscreens that do not block the entire spectrum of sun rays (ultraviolet A and B rays), zinc oxide creams physically prevent all sun rays from damaging your skin.

Prior to many recent innovations, zinc oxide creams were not widely used because a white or gray color remained on the skin after application. However, due to microtechnology, zinc oxide creams can now be rubbed into the skin to provide an invisible layer of protection.

See also: Free radicals, sun protection, sunscreen, titanium dioxide

	Over the Counter	Prescription	Procedure at Dr's. Office	Procedure at Spa*
Alexandrite laser			✓	
Alloderm			✓	
Alphahydroxy acids	✓	✓	✓	✓
Amniotic fluid	✓			
Antioxidants	✓			
Artecoll			✓	
Astringents	✓			
Autologen			✓	
Azelex		✓		
Beta glucan	✓			
Betahydroxy acids	✓		✓	
Bleaching cream	✓	✓		
Blue Peel			✓	
Botox			✓	
Breast implants			✓	
Breast lift			✓	
Buf-Puf	✓			
CO_2 laser			✓	
Camouflage	✓			
Cautery			✓	
Celex-C	✓			
Cheek implants			✓	
Chemical peels			✓	✓

*Procedure performed at spas can also include salons.

	Over the Counter	Prescription	Procedure at Dr's. Office	Procedure at Spa
Chin implants			✓	
Collagen			✓	
Dermabrasion			✓	
Dermalogen			✓	
Desiccation			✓	
DHEA	✓			
Diode laser			✓	
Electrolysis				✓
Erbium:Yag laser			✓	
Ethocyn	✓			
Exfoliators	✓	✓	✓	✓
Eyebrow lift			✓	
Eyelid surgery			✓	
Face-lift			✓	
Facial masks	✓			✓
Facials				✓
Fat removal			✓	
Fat transplantation			✓	
Fibrel			✓	
Glycolic acid	✓	✓	✓	✓
Gore-Tex			✓	
Hair transplantation			✓	
Hormone creams	✓	✓		

	Over the Counter	Prescription	Procedure at Dr's. Office	Procedure at Spa
Isolagen			✓	
Jessner's peel			✓	
Kinetin	✓			
Kogic acid	✓	✓		
Lactic acid	✓	✓		
Laser dermabrasion			✓	
Lasers			✓	
Lip enhancement			✓	
Liposuction			✓	
Melatonin	✓			
Moisturizers	✓			
Neodymium:Yag laser			✓	
Phenol peel			✓	
Placenta extract	✓			
Power peel			✓	✓
Pulse dye laser			✓	
Renova		✓		
Restylane			✓	
Retin-A		✓		
Retinol	✓	✓		
Ruby laser			✓	
Salicylic acid	✓		✓	
Sclerotherapy			✓	

	Over the Counter	Prescription	Procedure at Dr's. Office	Procedure at Spa
SoftForm			✓	
Sunscreen	✓			
TCA			✓	
Thigh creams	✓			
Titanium dioxide	✓			
Toners	✓			
Vitamin A	✓			
Vitamin B	✓			
Vitamin C	✓	✓		
Vitamin E	✓			
Vitamin K	✓	✓		
Waxing	✓			✓
Zinc oxide	✓			

This table shows how the remedies described in *The Dermatologist's Guide to Looking Younger* are available for use. Some remedies are available as both lower-strength, over-the-counter and higher, prescription-strength forms.